Alternative Health Care

Medicine, Miracle, or Mirage?

Alternative Health Care

Medicine, Miracle, or Mirage?

Michael S. Goldstein

 Temple University Press
PHILADELPHIA

Temple University Press, Philadelphia 19122
Copyright © 1999 by Temple University.
All rights reserved
Published 1999
Printed in the United States of America

⊗ The paper used in this publication
meets the requirements of American National Standard for
Information Sciences—Permanence of Paper for Printed
Library Materials, ANSI Z39.48-1984

Library of Congress Cataloging-in-Publication Data

Goldstein, Michael S., 1944–
    Alternative health care : medicine, miracle, or mirage? /
Michael S. Goldstein.
        p.   cm.
    ISBN 1-56639-677-8 (cloth : alk. paper). —
    ISBN 1-56639-678-6(pbk. : alk. paper)
    1. Alternative medicine—Social aspects—United States.
2. Alternative medicine—United States—Public opinion.
3. Public health—United States.   4. Holistic medicine.
5. Mind and body therapies.   I. Title
R733.G654   1999
615.5—DC21   98–27769
                                                      CIP

To my father, Abraham,
a man of strength and kindness

Contents

Acknowledgments

If not for Michael Ames, my editor at Temple University Press, this book would not have been written. He urged me to write the prospectus and showed me how to change it into something much better than it was.

The quality of what I've produced has been infinitely enhanced by two of the most wonderful research assistants. Sara Shostak worked with me in the early stages, assembling and shaping the raw material into a first draft. Her perceptiveness, intellectual acuity, and unfailing good spirits were crucial in too many ways to mention. Anna Dorman assisted me at the later stages, rewriting, editing, and preparing the manuscript. Her clarity, grace, and good judgment reflect those pervasive qualities within her.

I was able to pay these two assistants through the generosity of a grant from the Fetzer Institute of Kalamazoo, Michigan. The institute's support, and especially the support of the late Ken Klivington, was essential and is gratefully acknowledged.

1 The Emergence of Alternative Medicine

In 1983 when Joshua, my oldest son, was eighteen months old, a hot iron fell on his foot and remained there until the person watching him discovered it. Most of the skin on the top of his tiny foot was gone. The emergency room doctor, his pediatrician, and three or four physician friends who examined him all agreed this was a "third-degree burn." There was no way it could ever heal by itself. The only reasonable course of action was a skin graft. The well-known surgeon at a highly regarded burn center concurred. Laura (his mother) and I both felt lucky that the surgery could be scheduled very quickly. But our feelings changed when we found out that our son would have to be tied to his bed for the entire lengthy hospitalization to prevent him from scratching at the graft, and that the sight of this would be so upsetting that we would be restricted to a brief visit each day.

There had to be something else we could try before subjecting our little baby, no less ourselves, to such an ordeal. Laura's brother had a suggestion. He knew that in Japan, after the atomic bomb was dropped, the juice of the aloe vera plant had been used to treat people with much more severe burns. When we decided to try this ourselves, the Japanese proprietor of a nearby nursery offered helpful advice on which parts of the plant to use and how to start growing our own supply so as not to be dependent on him. Three times a day I carefully dripped the freshly cut aloe vera onto the wound. As I did, I drew on my

1

own knowledge about how imagery affects the body. I would speak to my son in a soothing voice, pointing his finger at his foot and describing over and over what I wanted to happen: "The white part of your skin at the edge is a tiny bit bigger than it was yesterday, the dark part is a tiny bit smaller. . . . Good, good. Your skin is getting stronger. Let's think about how the juice is helping your skin grow." In about three months the foot had healed. By the time Joshua was six, only the slightest outline of the burn could be detected.

As soon as it was clear that the burn had healed, Laura proposed that we get in touch with all the physicians who had advised a skin graft for our son. Surely they would want to know about a less intrusive and less costly alternative. Those we spoke with were all happy about the outcome. But not a single one was willing to say that they might suggest our solution to someone else in a similar predicament. It wasn't only their fear of a malpractice suit. Most were frank: treating a third-degree burn with aloe vera was just too far removed from what they had learned, and what their colleagues would find acceptable. Our experience, no matter how important for us, meant little or nothing to them.

By 1996, when I started to write this book, the situation was vastly different. In September of that year, a *Life Magazine* cover story, "The Healing Revolution," predicted that health care in America was about to be "completely transformed" by the integration of "ancient medicine and new science to treat everything from the common cold to heart disease." The first page featured a dramatic photograph of cardiac surgery being performed at New York City's Columbia-Presbyterian Hospital, with an "energy healer" laying on hands alongside the surgeon. Anyone who frequents a newsstand would hardly have been surprised to come upon this cover story. During the few months prior, stories about alternative medicine had appeared on the covers of both *Newsweek* and *Time*.

These prominent cover stories are but one manifestation of the immense amount of attention that the mass media have given to something that is variously referred to as "alternative medicine," "holistic medicine," or "complementary medicine." A visit to any large chain bookstore will reveal an abundance of books about alternative medicine; they fill the large sections devoted to health, medicine, self care, and self help. Just one of Deepak Chopra's books on alternative medicine, *Ageless Body, Timeless Mind: The Quantum Alternative to Growing Old,* has sold more than seven million copies since it was first published in 1993. Sales figures for this book and similar ones by physician-authors like Larry Dossey, Bernie Siegel, and Andrew Weil have consistently placed them atop the best seller lists. To the extent that the American public reads nonfiction books, they are likely to be about alternative medicine.

Some of the media attention and popular concern comes from the vivid personal testimony offered on behalf of various alternative treatments. Celebrity accounts have received a good deal of attention. Shirley Maclaine, who has abandoned Western medical pharmacology for "the healing powers to be found in acupuncture, spirit messages and crystal rocks," now teaches that we can all learn to heal ourselves by visualizing colors specific to each area of the body. The powerful description by cultural critic Norman Cousins of his battle with "an incurable illness," ankylosing spondylitis, was particularly influential. Cousins attributed his success in recovering from what doctors thought to be an irreversible illness to his alternative approach to healing. He reasoned that "if negative emotions produce negative chemical reactions in the body, wouldn't the positive emotions produce positive chemical changes?" On this basis he stopped his medication, checked himself out of the hospital, began an innovative regimen of massive doses of vitamin C and amusing movies, and sought "love, hope, faith, laughter, confidence, and the will to live. . . ." His successful recovery made him a crusader for his views. Since he was well connected and widely respected for his probing intellect, those who may have scoffed at the anecdotes of others were less likely to dismiss Cousins's story. Although his experience became widely known through his book, the initial account (upon which the book is based) appeared in the highly prestigious *New England Journal of Medicine* (*NEJM*) and included his assertion that "the hospital was no place for a person who was seriously ill." Cousins spent the remainder of his years on a medical school faculty trying to persuade academic medical researchers to take his ideas seriously.

Vivid stories detailing all sorts of personal battles and triumphs over life-threatening diseases through the use of alternative healing practices have become common. *Double Vision: An East-West Collaboration for Coping with Cancer* is among the most impressive. This book details how when twenty-one-year-old Drew Todd was diagnosed with a rare form of aggressive cancer, his mother Alexandra set out on an unrelenting quest to discover what was available beyond conventional care. Their story and similar accounts not only acquaint readers with many of the specific alternative techniques (Todd used a macrobiotic diet, relaxation, visualization, and acupuncture, among others), but deliver powerful messages about the possibility of personal transcendence and the shortcomings of the mainstream health care system.

For the most part, however, the media has paid attention to alternative medicine not merely because of the triumphs of the famous. Rather, a consistent stream of well-researched academic reports has emerged over the past several years, portraying the American population as actively engaged in alternative practices and as believing in the ideas that underlie many such techniques.

The most frequently cited of these accounts, a 1990 survey of a national sample of American adults, found that about one-third had used what was termed "unconventional medicine" in the past year to treat a medical problem. In 1997, when the researchers repeated the survey, those who reported using alternative therapies in the past year had jumped to over 42 percent. In both years affluent, highly educated whites were the most typical users. Although almost all the users of these unconventional techniques were using mainstream care at the same time, in both surveys over two thirds of the users did not discuss the unconventional therapy with their physician. The authors speculate that this "deficiency in patient-doctor relations" might "derive from medical doctors' mistaken assumption that their patients do not routinely use unconventional therapies for serious medical problems." Those who used unconventional treatments made an average of nineteen visits per year to "alternative providers" to receive care. By extrapolation the authors conclude that the 427 million visits Americans made to alternative practitioners in 1990 had grown by 47.3% to 629 million visits in 1997. This far exceeds the 336 million visits made to all primary care physicians that same year. The total out of pocket cost of all this alternative care was estimated to have increased by a similar proportion to more than 27 billion dollars in 1997, well in excess of what was spent out of pocket on all physician services. Yet the methodology of the study specifically excluded any visit or use of unconventional medicine for the purpose of prevention or health promotion, considered by many advocates to be the primary strengths of unconventional medicine. Therefore, these findings should be seen as very conservative estimates of the magnitude of the alternative medicine phenomenon. In fact, two other national surveys reported in 1998 also found that 42 percent of households polled had used some type of alternative care within the past year.

Research on specific forms of alternative care consistently presents a similarly impressive picture of extensive use. For example, approximately a third of all those who suffer from back pain—an extremely common, chronic condition—chose chiropractic rather than mainstream medicine for treatment. Depending on the study, between a quarter and a half of all individuals with a terminal illness seek alternative care at some point in the course of their disease. The prevalence of alternative medicine appears to be widespread regardless of the severity of the medical problem. Studies have indicated that socioeconomic status is either independent of the use of alternative medicine, or that higher status and more highly educated individuals are overrepresented among alternative medicine users.

Alternative health care is not always easy to define, however, or to distinguish from broader health promotion activities. This can make specific statistical findings difficult to interpret. For example, *Natural Foods Merchandiser* reports that sales of "natural foods" totaled $9.17 *billion* in 1995. But it is unclear how much of this sum can reasonably be considered to have been spent on alternative medicine. The $1.5 billion reported by the *Los Angeles Times* that Americans spent on "medicinal herbs" in that same year might be a better estimate, although to use this value assumes that we know how these herbs are being used. Thousands of people use "cat's claw" (a vine from the Amazon, long used by Peruvians for many types of healing) because they believe it will strengthen their immune systems. Are they practicing alternative medicine even if they are in good health? What if the user is HIV positive? Does using herbs for weight loss qualify as "alternative medicine"? Attempting to resolve these ambiguities leads to the matter of defining precisely what is meant by the term "alternative medicine," as well as the terms "prevention" and "cure," along with the most basic notions of "health" and "illness" themselves.

However these conceptual matters are resolved, the media, the public, policymakers, and many people in the established health professions have already begun to act in ways that break down whatever distinctions exist between alternative and conventional care. Just a few years ago, it would have been difficult to imagine an "energy healer" working side by side with a cardiac surgeon in the operating room at one of the nation's leading academic medical centers, much less the hospital allowing the scene to be photographed for *Life Magazine*. The growing trend of many health maintenance organizations (HMOs) to develop or "contract out" for "spiritual healing" programs could be dismissed as purely a marketing device, a public relations stunt, or even a cynical substitution of a very inexpensive form of care for one more costly. But a 1997 survey of three hundred HMO executives found that 94 percent believe personal prayer or other spiritual practices can aid medical treatment and accelerate healing. Recent reports have depicted numerous examples of conventional health care organizations recognizing alternative medicine. For example, in 1996 a panel of one hundred fourteen leading scientists and representatives of academia, drug companies, and community groups appointed by the National Institutes of Health (NIH) to review the nation's AIDS research effort issued a blistering report that recommends a greater focus on alternative medicine in future HIV/AIDS research. In the same year, Oxford Health Plan, which provides care to 1.4 million people in the eastern United States, announced that it would add alternative medicine to some of its health plans. The initial group assembled by Oxford included approximately one thousand chiropractors, acupuncturists, naturopathic doctors, massage therapists, and yoga instructors, with plans already underway to add practitioners of T'ai Chi and reflexology. In the wake of such reports, it is becoming increasingly difficult to ignore the possibility that a more fundamental change in society's orientation to health and healing is taking place.

Mainstream medicine's growing openness to various forms of alternative care is just beginning to have an impact on daily medical practice. In Europe, fairly high proportions of the established medical community either accept or practice alternative medicine to some degree. For example, in Britain about 40 percent of general practitioners state that they find homeopathy to be effective in some situations, and either refer clients or practice it themselves. In the United States, there has always been a small number of physicians who have practiced some form of alternative treatment. For the most part they have restricted their work to one or a few specific modes of treatment, and have been shunned by most other M.D.'s and the major medical organizations. Today, however, medical schools openly hold courses on many forms of alternative care, along with support groups for holistic and alternative physicians. There is even a national organization, the American Holistic Medical Association, that restricts its membership to M.D.'s and medical students.

By any measure of the number of people involved, money spent, professional regard, or public opinion, alternative medicine has taken on a significant and growing presence in America. Thus, it should be no surprise that the popular media are filled with news about alternative medicine. The national media have long given attention to developments in medicine and health care. Until recently, the media considered innovation and scientific or technical advances to be the essence of what was "newsworthy." It is striking, then, that the media, hundreds of newsletters, Internet sites, and other sources devoted to alternative medicine actually contain very little that is "new." The techniques and approaches to health and healing that are extolled (or condemned)—such as acupuncture, massage, homeopathy, chiropractic, naturopathy, and herbal medicine—are almost all therapeutic systems and modalities that have existed for hundreds or even thousands of years. Any long-time observer of alternative medicine in America would wonder, why this glut of attention *now*?

Understanding alternative medicine's position within the broader health care scene requires some description of how perceptions of health and health care among the general public and policymakers have changed over the past several decades. The successes and domination of "scientific" medicine have helped foster a climate of high costs, unreasonable expectations, distance, and distrust. These factors have combined with more longstanding critiques of the biomedical model of American health care to create what might be described as a popular "grievance" against Western medicine.

The career of Ralph Moss is a good example of how this "grievance" develops and interacts with the field of alternative medicine. Moss was a well-regarded science writer who eventually became assistant director of Public Affairs at the Sloan-Kettering Cancer Center in New York. His growing public disenchantment with the effectiveness of conventional cancer therapies, especially chemotherapy, led to his firing, and a new view of himself as a muckraking crusader whose articles and books like *The Cancer Industry* and *Questioning Chemotherapy* would give patients and their families an "insider's perspective." Over the past twenty years his writing has come to include more and more information about alternative cancer therapies, and he was asked to serve on the original advisory board of the federal government's Office of Alternative Medicine (OAM). Currently he supports himself by producing a regular journal on cancer therapy (*The Cancer Chronicles*) both in print and on-line, as well as reports on treatment options for people with cancer. He charges $275 each for each of these "Moss Reports."

The ambiguities that surround alternative medicine inhere in the term itself. Does "alternative medicine" indicate cohesion around some underlying conceptual framework, or is it merely a phrase of convenience? The popular media and many practitioners often speak of a "paradigm shift" or a "revolution" in understanding disease and healing. At the same time, other practitioners stress that alternative approaches can and should be integrated into mainstream health care. Is there truly a paradigm shift that underlies these techniques and approaches? If there is, what is it? If a "new paradigm" exists, can it coexist with mainstream doctors and hospitals, no less the rapidly changing health care system as it moves toward "managed care"? It seems clear that there *is* a coherent underlying set of commonalties that justifies viewing alternative medicine as a single, if broad and diverse, phenomenon. It would be a mistake to think of alternative medicine as merely a name for a residual list of techniques omitted from the standard medical school curriculum.

To find that alternative medicine is a conceptually coherent category does not necessarily imply that there is a corresponding empirical or organizational reality. There is no doubt that a plethora of professional associations, conferences, publications, support groups, and commercial enterprises devote themselves to "alternative medicine." But it is still not clear to what extent "alternative medicine" exists as an empirically verifiable social reality and how it relates to mainstream medicine. Do the people who practice some form of alternative medicine, and those who utilize some facet of it for real health problems, see it as a cohesive entity? The answer here is not at all clear-cut. However, an organizational reality increasingly is emerging and gaining acceptance among the public, the government, and the health care establishment. The extension of third-party insurance coverage to alternative therapies, the decision of some HMOs to develop networks of alternative medicine practitioners, and the opening of the Office of Alternative Medicine at the National Institutes of Health all indicate that the climate in the late 1990s is far more open to alternative medicine than it was just a few years ago.

The central role of religion and spirituality in many forms of alternative medicine is one factor that complicates the future of alternative medicine in America. Many health professionals have a difficult time accepting spirituality as a core component of health and healing. Understanding this tension is vital to predicting the future relationship between alternative and mainstream medicine.

Another potentially pivotal characteristic of alternative medicine is that it draws on ideologies associated with both the political "right" and "left," thereby transcending common political categories. Many of its basic criticisms of mainstream medicine emerge from a left perspective that opposes the dominance of professionals as well as excess profit-making in medicine. Alternative medicine also encompasses a strong countercultural component whose roots are on the left. Yet, the strong focus on enhanced individual responsibility for health, along with an emphasis on nongovernmental solutions to health problems, often gives alternative medicine a distinctly rightward cast. Examining a number of "political" struggles, such as the formation of the Office of Alternative Medicine at the National Institutes of Health and the efforts of alternative providers to gain licensure and third-party reimbursement, is the best way to understand the relationship of various political ideologies to alternative medicine.

Mainstream medicine in the United States is being fundamentally altered by nationwide efforts to hold down the costs of care and increase corporate control (usually referred to as "managed care"). In addition, there is ongoing debate about the escalating cost of health care to the government. These developments have significant implications for the future of alternative medicine. Both contain the potential for fostering its integration into the broader health care system and imposing restraints on the form and content of that integration. Any predictions about the future of alternative medicine will need to keep this new economic context in mind.

There is ample evidence that alternative medicine is assuming a greater role in the currents of American life. This will no doubt require more interaction, if not cooperation, with the medical mainstream, bringing with it the potential for cooptation and assimilation of that which is truly distinctive. The powerful economic forces changing mainstream medicine will likely exacerbate this possibility. At the same time, alternative medicine may be developing into an "identity movement" that offers a new understanding of what is possible both to its adherents and to society at large.

Today my son Joshua is a teenager with no real memory of his badly burned foot or of how it healed. His injury and recovery in 1983 has become only one of the many stories all families tell about themselves. It has much in common with the story the Todd family tells about Drew's cancer, and the stories Ralph Moss, Deepak Chopra, Andrew Weil, and many others offer their readers. All of these stories suggest that with some knowledge and effort you can harness the resources to triumph over much illness, suffering, and disability. This is a powerful message.

2 Victims of Medicine

To what is "alternative medicine" an alternative? In the United States health care institutions and professionals exist in such great numbers and diversity that defining what is meant by "mainstream" medicine is an increasingly difficult undertaking. In what observers call the "medicalization of everything," medical terms, workers, and institutions have come to encompass most every domain of human interaction. Given such profusion, defining mainstream medicine as that which is typically taught in medical schools and practiced in hospitals may seem reasonable.

In fact, mainstream medicine is undergoing constant change. Over the past few decades its credibility and status in society have been repeatedly challenged. Taken together, these challenges have fueled a search for new ways of understanding the nature of illness and of delivering health care. Alternative medicine is one response to this crisis in conventional care. Typically, the conceptual basis for delineating the medical mainstream is the notion that it is roughly synonymous with "scientific medicine," also frequently called "biomedicine." It is the dominance of scientific medicine and its elaboration in research, clinical practice, and the development of medical technology and specialties that comprise the medical mainstream.

Scientific medicine in America is usually traced to the reforms of the Flexner Report of 1910. The explicit goals of the Flexner Report, as well as the Carnegie Foundation that sponsored it and the small elite of European trained physicians who avidly supported it, were both to establish empirical scientific rationality as the basis of future medical training and practice in the United States and to dismiss any other form of medicine as nonscientific, and hence, illegitimate. Although the precise premises of "scientific medicine" were nowhere set out, they were fairly clear and have remained so: *Our bodies exist in an objective physical world. Each person's body is an entity unto itself, connected to others only by the physical aspects of genetic transmission. Although thoughts and emotions are likely to have a biophysical reality in the brain, the mind (and/or soul) of the individual is fundamentally separate from the body. The body is best understood mechanistically through the methods of laboratory science and experimentation, which are largely free of bias and the best means of discovering "truth."* The development and progressive domination of mainstream scientific medicine cannot be understood without an appreciation of the importance and (perceived) success of these premises as a means of comprehending and manipulating the natural world.

Despite the overwhelming dominance of this "scientific perspective" in medicine as it developed after Flexner, other ways of understanding the meaning and origins of health and illness persisted. These "alternative" views were often associated with specific healing techniques, such as acupuncture or herbalism. Sometimes they were connected to spiritual or religious movements such as Christian Science or Seventh Day Adventism. What most of these perspectives have in common is a rejection of the "objective" and physically knowable world as the sole locus of the sources of illness. The body is understood not as a machine, reducible to its constituent parts, but "holistically," as a system that is fully integrated and interpenetrating. While each of these specific approaches to illness has had its own views and language to explain the origins of health and illness, they have all held certain fundamental beliefs in common. These core beliefs are described in the next chapter. However, advocates of these alternative forms of healing were not the only groups in society to hold these views. In at least three respects, major currents of American intellectual life have been developing along lines that also conflict with the dominant perspective of post-Flexner, "scientific" medicine.

Changing Views of Health and Illness
Mind and Body

A central tenet of views critical of "scientific medicine" has been the overriding importance of the interconnectedness of mind and body. Scientific medicine's roots in the dualism of Descartes has precluded it from viewing the human being as an organic whole. This has led to the neglect, minimizing, and denial of the mind's ability to produce and remove symptoms, if not create and cure illness. The opposing "holistic" view starts with the assumption that an organism (the whole) is more than the sum of its parts. According to this perspective, the nature of the parts is determined by the whole with each part understandable only as an interdependent part of the whole. While the dominant views in medical education and practice since Flexner have given short shrift to holism, developments in psychology, laboratory science, epidemiology, physics, and many other fields did not.

The development of psychology as a field of inquiry and clinical practice exemplifies this gap with medicine. The work of many notable psychologists from John Dewey to Freud and the gestalt psychologists such as Wolfgang Kohler and Kurt Koffka, as well as the "human potential" psychologists such as Abraham Maslow, all viewed the human being as an indivisible unit of mind and body. The essence of living, and in particular the potential or overall goal-directed nature of the organism, could not be understood unless one comprehended this unity. While each of their perspectives influenced the development of American psychology, their work extended beyond the academic and clinical realms. This has been especially true of Maslow's theories, which directly led to the development of the "human potential movement" by Carl Rogers and others. The human potential movement was instrumental in carrying the message of holism to the fields of education, management, and organizational development, as well as to the worlds of art and music during the 1960s. Thus, psychology has been influential in contributing to holistic ideas about the interpenetration of mind and body and establishing them among the public, especially among the most educated and accomplished.

The growing recognition and understanding of the "placebo effect" has contradicted views that proclaim the mind and body as fundamentally separate. The placebo effect occurs when substances lacking intrinsic actions produce cures, distinguishing them from the results of "real" treatments. Although many mainstream clinicians had long recognized that part of their power to heal people derived from the symbolism and expectations both patients and practitioners brought to the therapeutic encounter, the formal recognition of that fact by medical educators and organized medicine was consistently downplayed. Remission of symptoms and cures lacking a "scientific" rationale could be dismissed as being "only the placebo effect." Mainstream practitioners have often trivialized the placebo effect, not because a suffering patient would reject being cured on that basis, but because it undermines the rational scientific approach of Western medicine. As Linnie Price put it, "The implications of the placebo effect for medicine, then, is that it relocates healing in the realm of the irrational. . . . If the pharmaceutical industry were able to produce a drug which was as reliable, of such wide-ranging applicability, and with a record of efficacy as impressive as that of the placebo effect, it would no doubt be proclaimed as a miracle panacea and attributed to the wonders of science."

Despite scientific medicine's ideological discomfort with the placebo effect, it has been the subject of much cross-cultural research as well as a topic of interest to a small number of physicians, who have described its omnipresence in every sort of medical encounter from psychotherapy to surgery. Placebos have been shown to effectively treat a wide variety of conditions, including mood changes, angina pectoris, headache, seasickness, anxiety, hypertension, depression, and the common cold. Placebos can work for years, reducing symptoms as long as the patient believes them to be "real." Additionally, placebos have been shown to mimic the effect of active pharmacological agents and to be capable of producing many of the formal traits of drug dependency. Moreover, several studies have chronicled negative side effects in patients being treated with placebos and indicated that "just as a belief that a placebo is a 'real' drug produced a 'real' effect, belief that a real drug is a placebo produces a lack of effect." These studies provide evidence that the placebo effect remains as powerful as ever in the age of "scientific medicine."

Ironically, it was the cumulative efforts of medical researchers, most of whom wished to demonstrate the efficacy of a new drug or technique, that provided the strongest testimony of the prominence and prevalence of the placebo effect. According to the standards of Western scientific medicine, "proof" of the efficacy of a new drug or technique requires the use of so-called "double blind" randomized controlled trails. By using random assignment to determine whether study participants will receive either a treatment drug or a placebo, and keeping both the participant and the clinician ignorant of which subjects have received which treatments, this type of study design is considered the most rigorous means of ascertaining the "true" effect of the drug being evaluated. This approach to medical research explicitly minimized the usefulness of clinical reports of success. The entire methodology was based upon the premise that if either the doctor or the patient (no less both) knew which treatment was "supposed to" work, it would indeed succeed. The working assumption in medical research was that the placebo effect was an overriding presence, in constant need of being excluded if any sense was to be made

of proposed innovations. Yet despite this omnipresent acknowledgment of the placebo effect's ubiquity and power, little attention was given to how its impact might be enhanced for the
benefit of patients, much less what it implied about the underlying assumptions concerning the relation of body and mind.

In like fashion, the critique of classical physics arising from
the development of "the new physics" has raised questions
about the adequacy of the current scientific biomedical model.
The new physics refers to the theories of quantum mechanics,
based on Max Planck's theory of quanta in 1900, and relativ-
ity, which began with Albert Einstein's special theory of rela-
tivity in 1905. According to the new physics, a complete understanding of reality lies beyond the capabilities of rational
thought, and, at best, physics can merely describe the statistical behavior of systems and predict probabilities. That is to
say, the new physics contravenes positivism, disputing the possibility of a detached and objective science in pursuit of "absolute truth." Indeed, Bell's Theorem, a keystone of the new
physics, posits that "underneath" ordinary space-time phenomena, there lies a deep nonlocal reality in which none of the
"laws" of classical physics apply. Moreover, the new physics
insists that it is not possible to observe reality without changing it; there is no objective reality apart from our experience.
Therefore, our experience of the event occurs at the moment
we observe the event. This implies that our experience of reality is determined by our own consciousness. Thus, these developments in physics question the validity of the assumptions
upon which conventional scientific medicine is based. Additionally, they transcend traditional views which hold that mental and physical phenomena are functionally different.

Health and Community

Biologists have long noted that all species, plant or animal, live
in communities. Existence apart from others for any extensive

length of time is rare and usually futile. Literature, anecdotal commentary, and scores of research reports have set out the consequences of social isolation for the physical health of humans. Anthropologists have described the rapid onset of death in members of small tribal groups who are ostracized, and numerous contemporary statistical accounts show the impact of bereavement upon the short-term mortality rates of those who survive. A typical finding in this literature is that about 20 percent of those who die within a year after the death of their spouse do so in direct physiologic response to the psychological impact of the loss. Scientists have demonstrated the physiological mechanism by which loneliness and isolation lead to poor physical health among primates, and it is generally thought to operate similarly in humans. Recently, a large study of nine hundred forty-two Finnish men found that feelings of hostility, hopelessness, and cynicism sharply accelerated atherosclerosis in carotid arteries, a major precursor to stroke.

Since the 1960s a large body of rigorous research has demonstrated how job-related stress can adversely affect one's health. In 1973, *Work in America: Report of a Special Task Force to the Secretary of Health, Education and Welfare* found that dissatisfaction with one's work was the single best predictor of a heart attack—superior to blood pressure, cholesterol, or any other traditional "risk factor." Subsequent research has been able to specify those particular job characteristics that lead to especially high risk, such as limited decision-making ability coupled with high job demands. Researchers have also identified certain job characteristics that are protective against heart attacks, such as feelings of control and commitment. Large epidemiologic studies, carried out in Britain, have clearly shown the relationship of the type of job one holds in the occupational hierarchy to be related to most major causes of death, independent of risk factors like smoking and blood pressure, or of access to medical care.

This research has not primarily focused on the health of

individuals in a clinical context. Rather, these studies have dealt with the health of populations and groups. However, the findings from these population-based community studies suggest associations that are similar to the results of the more individually-focused psychological work on social isolation described earlier. Common to both approaches is an emphasis on the interpenetration of the mental and the physical realms of life. Social relationships and events can either create distress and literally make someone sick, or relieve distress and make someone well. Health and illness exist as points on a continuum, in a constantly changing relationship to each other. Resources for maintaining health or fighting illness may exist in an individual's environment, but they must be perceived as beneficial if they are to be effective. It is perceived meaning, our thoughts, derived from the sum total of our life experience that determines our propensity to be healthy or ill. The implication of all this work is clear: the communal environment, which includes our relationships with other people, enters our bodies via the symbols and categories in our minds. As in the development of social psychology and in the studies of the placebo effect, the essence of this research is that the line between our selves and those around us is blurred. Thus, a basic tenet of the "medical" view of illness is undermined. As in the case of the placebo effect, despite having been conducted under the auspices of medical institutions, this research has had only a minimal impact on clinical practice.

Regardless of conventional medicine's neglect of these ideas about the interpenetration of mind, body, and the community, such notions are quite compatible with the views held by most forms of Judeo-Christian religion, as well as various types of Eastern, "new age," and humanistic spiritual groups. The former have always been an important force within American life. The latter have come to play an increasingly significant role as the population has become more ethnically diverse, more highly educated, and more secular. Although the major religions have been very receptive towards mainstream scientific medicine, each encompasses a tradition that stresses the potential of body-mind interaction and the importance of the relationship between the suffering patient and healer, along with the connection between the individual and the community as both a source of sickness and healing. To the extent that religion and spirituality have provided a counterpoint to the dominant American values of scientific rationalism, they have also offered an alternative to scientific biomedicine for understanding health and healing. The recent ascendancy of charismatic, Pentecostal, and "born again" movements within American Christianity has greatly enlarged the number of people who know about and accept some alternative views of how healing may occur.

Many Americans have become familiar with a quasi-religious perspective on healing through their contact with 12-step programs and other self-help groups. Modeled on the premises of Alcoholics Anonymous, 12-step programs require turning oneself over to a "higher power" as a condition of help or healing. Robert Wuthnow, a professor of sociology at Princeton University, estimates that there are approximately three million spiritually oriented self-help groups in the United States, many in churches and others based on the 12-step framework. The twenty-year-old New Age movement has also had a significant impact on Americans' spiritual beliefs. Respected public opinion polls repeatedly find that belief in various forms of "alternative realities" is common and positively associated with education. At least half the adult population admits to a belief in the existence of angels, and in the period between 1990 and 1995, over two hundred books concerned with the topic of angels have been published. The World Wide Web boasts approximately three thousand mystically-oriented sites.

Even physicians are joining the ranks of those who believe that there is a role for spirituality in healing. According to a 1996 statement released by the Harvard Medical School, over

99 percent of the three hundred family physicians interviewed by an independent research firm reported that they "believe in the ability of religious beliefs to contribute positively to the healing process." Additionally, 80 percent of the surveyed physicians believe in the "palliative powers of meditation and prayer," and 55 percent reported that they use relaxation and meditation techniques in their practice.

This widespread prevalence of groups proclaiming and promoting a spiritual or religious dimension to healing as well as the rise and ubiquity of 12-step programs reflects and reinforces beliefs about health and illness that are fundamentally at odds with the traditional biomedical worldview.

Prevention versus Curing

Since its earliest days, Western medicine has encompassed a range of views about how a state of health is best achieved. Dubos describes the "competition" between the Greek gods Hygeia and Asclepius. Hygeia represented the possibility of preventing or forestalling illness by living in a healthy manner, what today would be called "health promotion." Asclepius, the first physician according to Greek legend, achieved fame not by teaching wisdom but by "the use of the knife and the bandage of curative plants." There is little doubt that Asclepius's approach became the dominant view of medicine. Today his image and name are frequently represented on medical institutions. However, the views of Hygeia did not disappear completely. Those seeking the "laws" of a healthy life, the prevention of illness, and the building of healthy communities maintained a presence within medicine, most commonly under the rubric of "public health." Although this catchall term has, for many, become synonymous with the units of state and local government that bear the name, the field is much broader. As seen in schools of public health (which originally were restricted to the post-graduate training of physicians and other health professionals), public health includes the assessment and measurement of community health, prevention of illness, and effects of environmental factors on human health, along with the administrative dimension of health care. In many respects public health schools and agencies have served as a refuge on the border of mainstream medicine for health providers working to improve the health of communities.

Despite its marginalized status, public health research has consistently documented the limited role that clinical medicine and medical technology have played in reducing mortality in industrialized nations. Public health research has also provided evidence of the crucial roles played by social status, working conditions, the physical environment, and social relationships in promoting health. Removed from its bureaucratic and professional "home" in public health schools and agencies, the underlying message of public health is strikingly similar to the views held by other critics of mainstream medicine: *Health is a product of community life which reflects social distinctions and hierarchies and is modifiable by environmental change and alteration in the way in which people relate to each other.* Aggressive calls for the primacy of a "public health paradigm"—or a "biopsychosocial model"—over the dominant biomedical model have recently become relatively common among public health leadership. After-the-fact clinical interventions are seen as a diversion from the goal of preventing illness. In the case of problems such as chronic illness, substance abuse, and mental illness, prevention is heavily dependent upon changes in the consciousness, or the "empowerment" of people and groups.

The congruencies and convergence among public health advocates, psychologists documenting mind-body interaction, and social scientists charting the influence of the community on health are striking. Although many commentators such as Rick Carlson, Ivan Illich, and Irving Zola noted the intersecting lines of thought and saw the potential affinity between them, these critics of conventional biomedicine have carried on their work independently of each other. Yet despite their relative infrequency and isolation, these criticisms of mainstream medicine have become increasingly influential. The heightened prominence, synergy, and impact of these critiques have not been due to any newfound validity as much as to their affinity with a wholly distinct set of changes in the mainstream medical care system.

Crisis and Change in the Health Care System

Since the late 1960s, health care in the United States has commonly been described as being in a state of "crisis," "transformation," or "flux." While the specifics of what constituted a "crisis" varied widely, academics, journalists and politicians came to agree that we were embarking upon a period of major and significant change.

Contemporary portrayals of the changes taking place in health care range from the highly optimistic to the very pessimistic. Most of the optimism derives from hoped-for advances in the techniques of care. The public expectantly awaits genetic interventions, improvements in surgical techniques, or new vaccines. But it has generally viewed the ongoing and rapidly accelerating changes in the organization of health care more ambivalently, if not ominously. This fearful or pessimistic view of the evolution of our health care system can be traced to many sources, with a wide range of opinions about which factors have primacy. However, the key elements, regardless of their relative import, are well agreed upon.

The problem most frequently cited is simply the cost of health care to the society as a whole. In 1960 the United States spent well under 6 percent of its gross domestic product on medical care. By 1989 that proportion had doubled, and by 1994 it was just under 14 percent, where it has remained since. The 4.4 percent growth in health care spending for 1996 was the smallest percent change in over thirty years, but still about

25 percent above the overall rise in the gross domestic product. In absolute terms this expenditure exceeded $1 trillion for health care in 1996, or $3,759 a person. Even with such immense outlays, about forty-two million Americans have absolutely no health insurance coverage. While 99.7 percent of those aged sixty-five and older have coverage via Medicare or some other federally subsidized program, about 22 percent of those between the ages of sixteen and twenty-five have no health insurance at all. A 1996 report from the Census Bureau found that 38.2 percent of the Hispanic population and 30.1 percent of the Black population lacked health insurance for at least some portion of a twenty-eight-month period ending in August 1994, compared to 21.0 percent of Whites. No one is pleased by these figures.

Not surprisingly, the majority of money is spent on individuals who are ill. Medical services for those who are the most sick, who also tend to be the oldest and most likely to be covered by insurance, account for a disproportionate amount of health care expenditures. Those with chronic conditions account for about three-quarters of all the nation's health care costs. Ten percent of all Medicare recipients account for 70 percent of the program's outlays. The aging of the American population can only exacerbate these spending patterns. For example, the expected rapid growth among the "oldest old," those aged eighty-five and above, is projected to yield a 600 percent increase in Medicare costs by the year 2040 when the surviving "baby boomers" reach that age. In that same year, the number of nursing home residents over eighty-five years of age is expected to be about three times the total of today's entire nursing home population.

Concern regarding health care costs goes well beyond their absolute magnitude. In the United States, a higher percentage of total costs is devoted to administrative costs than in other industrialized nations, and these costs are growing. Despite widespread attention and concern, it appears that the health care system is becoming more inefficient. The current emphasis on managed care and converting nonprofit facilities and insurers, such as Blue Cross, into proprietary operations has heightened this trend. Administrative costs, profit, and costly high technology interventions for those most ill, often during the last few months of life, have been consuming ever larger shares of the nation's total health care expenses.

Given the immense amounts of money involved, much of it flowing directly or indirectly from government coffers, it is surprising how little evidence there is that greater expenditures for medical care produce better health or more healing. Although some researchers have argued that there is a marginal gain in the health status of the population in an industrialized nation when expenditures for medical care go up, most economists, epidemiologists, and others have been more skeptical.

The proportion of the national gross domestic product spent on health care has been of more interest to politicians, policymakers, and academics than to the average citizen. The typical patient is more concerned with the changing manner in which care has come to be provided. The decade after 1985 saw a massive change in the organization of American medicine in the form of the rise of "managed care." Simply put, this means that large for-profit corporations have become responsible for a growing share of health care services. By 1993, a majority of Americans who were privately insured were in managed care plans that restricted their choice of physicians. Large employers were the leaders in promoting this trend; 65 percent of their employees were covered under managed care plans. The most common form of managed care, the HMO or health maintenance organization, was fast transforming from what was a traditionally nonprofit organization, into a profit-making corporation. Managed care companies themselves were engaged in rapid consolidation. Mergers and acquisitions among managed care plans for the years 1993 and 1994 were valued at about $38 billion, and the rate and value of joint ventures has increased since that time.

Medicine is no longer largely a cottage industry of small providers (typically individual physicians) who interact through professional organizations and informal networks, sometimes coordinate their work in hospitals, and receive compensation on a piecework basis from both clients and insurance companies. Increasingly, physicians work for large profit or nonprofit corporations under contracts that subject them to detailed oversight, restrict their ability to exercise clinical judgement, and offer financial incentives to limit or skew the services they provide as a means of enhancing corporate profit. Managed care companies behave just like any other large corporation. Medicine is now "big business" and health care is a commodity.

It is not necessary here to judge whether managed care is a good or bad thing for the quality of American health care, or the health of the American population. A large quantity of both popular and academic literature has already emerged on that topic. What is clear is that the overall environment in which many, if not most, Americans receive their health care has shifted dramatically. Traditional arrangements and relationships between patients, physicians, hospitals, and insurers have all been changed in such a way as to limit long-term involvement, heighten distrust, and make medicine less "special" for all parties. The sense that health care is a commodity like any other is far more widespread and influential today than at any other time in the past. In addition to these broad changes in the organization of health care, and its rising cost to the nation, there is a growing mood of disenchantment with medicine. A number of recent polls report the public's growing dissatisfaction with managed care. Over half of Americans surveyed in a 1997 Lou Harris Poll felt managed care was actually harmful to their health.

What doctors do, and how well they do it, has emerged as a matter of attention and concern in the minds of clients, policymakers, and the general public. A notable but typical example is the controversy regarding the treatment and prevention of breast cancer, which has been highly publicized in recent years.

Initially, disputes emerged when data from trials conducted under the supervision of the National Cancer Institute suggested that lumpectomy (surgical removal of the tumor) followed by radiation treatment was as effective in treating breast cancer as mastectomy. These findings suggested that thousands of women had undergone unnecessary body-altering surgery. However, confidence in the enterprise of medical research itself was undermined seriously in April 1994 when the *Chicago Tribune* reported that one of the participating research physicians had falsified information about the patients he entered in the lumpectomy study, as well as those in a concurrent study, on the use of tamoxifen, a drug used in hormone therapy for breast cancer survivors. Though the falsifications did not influence the outcomes of the study, both the occurrence of the fraud and the fact that project administrators had not disclosed it in the more than four years in which they had known of its occurrence contributed enormously to popular disenchantment with the medical establishment.

The public's confusion about breast cancer was heightened in 1997, when the guidelines for using mammography to detect breast cancer in asymptomatic women in their forties became the subject of ongoing debate. The official recommendations of national institutions such as the American Cancer Society and the National Cancer Institute had changed no less than six times during the proceeding few years. Therefore, at the request of the National Cancer Institute, the NIH convened a panel of experts to evaluate existing data and determine mammography guidelines for women younger than fifty years of age. As is common practice when research findings are confusing, the panel reached its decision through a "consensus conference."

Traditionally, the conclusions of such conferences are so highly valued that they are used by insurance companies to determine benefits and by doctors and hospitals to determine standards of care. However, when the mammography panel announced its findings, both the health sector and the public responded with outrage. Neither group wanted to accept the panel's conclusion that "at the present time the available data do not warrant a single recommendation for mammography for all women in their forties. Each woman should decide for herself whether to undergo mammography." The director of the National Cancer Institute, Dr. Richard Klausner, at whose behest the panel was convened, said he was "shocked" and noted that an advisory board to the National Cancer Institute would review the decision the next month. The American Cancer Society issued a statement saying that it was "disappointed" in the report and stood by its recommendation that women in their forties have regular mammograms. One radiologist said he believed that the panel's actions were "tantamount to a death sentence" for women in their forties and that he "grieved for them." Another radiologist from the Harvard School of Medicine called the report "fraudulent" and admonished that it should not be released to the public until it was "corrected." The panel stood by its findings, noting that the data indicates 98.5 percent of women who get mammograms in their forties receive no benefit and that mammography carries risks of its own, including falsely telling women that there might be a tumor present, treating as cancerous a tiny lump that might or might not be cancerous but would require treatment if it were cancer, and giving women a false sense of security. Members of the panel also characterized the reactions to their report as "scary," and the chairman of the panel noted that "the arguments have gotten so strident that people are unwilling to listen."

Some analysts have explained the intensity of the reaction by noting that mammography is a big business in the United States. Others have commented that mammography has been widely promoted to women as a preventive measure that can save them from a dreaded disease, a reassurance and sense of protection with which women are reluctant to part. However, a more basic concern is that when the leading experts disagree so vehemently on how breast cancer should be diagnosed and treated, it raises basic questions about whom the public can trust. While the health issues brought up in the breast cancer and mammography controversies are highly specific, and of greatest concern to only a portion of the population, they are typical of many similar examples. Taken together, the frequency and intensity of such conflicts have abetted the broader decline in confidence about medicine in general.

The outpouring of concern about specific medical procedures and practices is, in some large measure, due to the rise in health care costs and discontent about the changing organization of care. Those factors have been central in motivating government and insurance companies to begin evaluating more precisely where their money is going. Increasingly the government and the insurance industry have been funding and carrying out research, varyingly called "health services research," "evaluation research," and "outcomes research," in order to get "hard data" (i.e., statistical evidence, as opposed to clinical reports) about a vast array of clinical procedures and tests. Almost inevitably, the data supports their initial concerns that the interventions are ineffective or overused, fostering still more concern and research.

The results of research on medical techniques, judgement, and practices heightens the public's mistrust about mainstream medicine in a number of ways. For example, in the United States *each year,* over 2 percent of all women have hysterectomies— a rate almost ten times as high as it is for women in France. This finding is typical of repeated demonstrations that regional and national political boundaries strongly influence the utilization of specific medical procedures, even when the incidence of a problem is similar. Results like this, along with research specifying the personal and idiosyncratic factors physicians use in deciding who to treat or what new procedures to adopt, causes clinical decision-making to appear more a matter of social norms and values than of the objective application of rationality.

Most unsettling for mainstream medicine has been the repeated finding that many "standard" medical procedures and therapies are of limited value, or even harmful. The culturally cherished "annual physical exam" for adults has been revealed as having no use in the screening for asymptomatic illness. A report in the *Journal of the American Medical Association* (*JAMA*) found that the widely publicized and heavily promoted PSA (prostate specific antigen) screening exam for prostate cancer leads to "a net health harm rather than a net health benefit." *NEJM* published a report concluding that it may be pure coincidence that people with chronic back pain, the second most common reason for visiting a physician, have disc abnormalities. The same prestigious journal reported that experienced board certified radiologists disagreed more than 20 percent of the time when reading mammograms on whether a biopsy should be performed. One study found that the medical records of 60 percent of elderly people admitted to the hospital failed to list the important medications being taken. A review of over thirty thousand randomly selected medical records from acute care hospitals in New York found 4 percent of the patients seriously injured by their treatment. More than 13 percent of these injuries led to death. A study by the American Hospital Association estimated that in 1983, 7 percent of all hospital admissions (approximately 2.7 million admissions in that year) were related to the misuse of pharmaceuticals prescribed by physicians and that such drug-induced illnesses cost up to $5 billion. A 1998 meta-analysis published in *JAMA* suggested that even when drugs are used properly, adverse reactions kill more than one hundred thousand Americans each year. The significance of these examples lies not in the "facts" they report. Rather, they are important because they represent a large and growing universe of similar findings in the medical literature and because each of them, along with numerous others, received prominent coverage in the popular media.

Conflicts, ambiguities, and failures of modern medicine,

along with news of "magic bullets" and medical heroism, are a regular part of the news in the 1990s. Cover stories in national magazines, front-page stories in the daily paper, and reports on radio and TV are commonly devoted to the sorts of critical findings cited above. This media attention indicates how important detailed information about health and medicine has become in our collective awareness. Yet often, the substance and tone of what is reported can only raise the consumer's level of skepticism, distance, and distrust. When medical researchers criticize their colleagues for *undertreating* pain and ignoring the evidence on how well pain medications work if used properly, while the chief medical writer for the *Los Angeles Times* gives major coverage to the *overuse* of pain medication and the resulting need for patients to "tolerate discomfort," the underlying message to the general public is one of confusion.

Ironically, it is the application of the scientific method to study the effectiveness of medical care that has yielded the intellectual power and empirical analyses which inspire doubt in mainstream "scientific" medicine itself. Observers inside and outside of the medical profession have long commented upon how little of what is considered standard treatment has any documented scientific basis showing it is indeed efficacious. In 1978, a report from the Congressional Office of Technology Assessment indicated that only 10 to 20 percent of all procedures currently used in medical practice had been shown to work in clinical trials. There has been little, if any, improvement since that time. Yet until recently, these research findings have had minimal impact on the public and policymakers. Despite the equivocal evidence, scientific rationality and the practice of medicine have been inextricably linked in the public mind.

As the dominance of the medical profession has grown and the expense of medical care burgeoned, the government, insurers, and industry (who foot the bills for most care) have become much more interested in knowing how much rational basis actually exists for the expenses they incur. It has become common for federal agencies such as the National Institutes of Health, the Health Care Financing Agency, and the Agency for Health Care Policy Research, as well as private foundations and "think tanks" such as Rand, to rely on randomized clinical trials, outcome evaluations, and epidemiological research to judge the true value of medical tests and procedures. Those who fund and carry out this research have been quite aggressive in publicizing their findings to the medical profession and the general public. Their predominantly negative or, at best, equivocal conclusions have helped foster and legitimize skepticism toward conventional medicine among policymakers and the general public.

Beyond its own intrinsic merit, the outcome of this research has an affinity with a number of other streams of academic thought that have been critical of medicine and the medical profession, such as "labeling theory" in sociology, and "attribution theory" in psychology. These perspectives emphasize the way in which the words we use shape our reactions to phenomena in the world. Both perspectives have stressed the ways in which "medical names" for signs, symptoms, conditions, and behaviors can highly stigmatize the individuals to whom they are applied. Researchers have found this to be especially true in regard to disabilities, physical illnesses like AIDS, and mental illnesses such as schizophrenia.

This extensive criticism of medicine has had a broad impact upon society. Analysts and policymakers have come to sharply divergent conclusions. Some view the epidemiologic and health service research as reason for some sort of national health care restructuring based upon federal insurance and increased government involvement in medicine. Others have come to a very different conclusion, arguing that the best policies are those which treat health care as any other commodity in the marketplace.

Individuals, especially those most economically secure and highly educated, have heightened their skepticism about the medical profession and have developed a high degree of "consumerism" toward medical care. Consumer publications such as *Consumer Reports* magazine and other media directed toward general audiences, such as "lifestyle" sections of many daily newspapers, have begun to report in detail about all sorts of medical and surgical techniques. Much of this material offers "user friendly" summaries of health services evaluations and outcomes research. These popular accounts have encompassed the widest range of medical interventions, including many that emerge from alternative approaches. Typical examples include the use of beta carotene in preventing heart disease and cancer, spinal manipulation as a treatment for back pain, herbal remedies to relieve depression, diet and relaxation techniques to reduce blood pressure, and melatonin for just about everything. Each of these summaries is consistent in noting that regardless of the specific topic being considered, medical experts disagree.

This combination of skepticism (sometimes carrying over into overt hostility) toward mainstream medicine and consumerism has become an important dimension of a number of social movements. The women's movement, the gay liberation movement, and movements for the rights of the disabled, chronically ill, and abused all have stressed that a medically dominated understanding of their members' problems is usually not helpful, and that medical solutions to these problems are highly questionable. The gay and lesbian communities' extensive advocacy for the declassification of homosexuality as an "illness" is one of the best examples of a successful challenge to a medically dominated characterization of a group of people. The women's movement has advocated for the reconceptualization of birth as a natural process, not a "medical condition," and the hospice movement has sought to redefine death and dying.

Skepticism about medicine is one element all of these movements hold in common. These individuals and groups do not deny that medicine may have much that they need or desire.

Rather, they wish to carefully evaluate what medicine has to offer, instead of uncritically accepting medical explanations for their problems and medical strategies for their improvement. They want to use medicine on their own terms. They are acutely aware that in the past medicine has harmed minorities and women in their quest for both individual and collective advancement. This outlook is epitomized by *The New Our Bodies, Ourselves,* the best selling health manual of the women's movement. In the book's chapter entitled "The Politics of Women and Medical Care," the authors cite "thousands" of personal accounts of the harm done to women by physicians and other medical personnel in medical settings who have:

> not listened to them or believed what they said; withheld knowledge, lied to them, treated them without their consent; not warned of risks and negative effects of treatment; overcharged them; experimented on them . . . ; treated them poorly because of their race, sexual preference, age, or disability; offered them tranquilizers or moral advice instead of medical care or useful help from community resources . . . ; administered treatments which were unnecessarily mutilating and too extreme for their problem, or which resulted in permanent disability or even death; prescribed drugs which hooked them, sickened them, changed their entire lives; performed operations which they later found were unnecessary, and removed organs which were in no way diseased; and abused them sexually.

The New Our Bodies, Ourselves debunks as "myth" popular ideas about the superiority of the American medical system, the contributions of medicine to world health, the scientific basis of medicine, the safety and efficacy of medical treatments, and the role of medicine in promoting health. Furthermore, the authors explicitly critique the medical system as an instrument for the social control and suppression of women. One outgrowth or manifestation of this skepticism is an openness to alternative approaches, as exemplified in the introduction to the book which states that while "we *do* need professional help with health problems . . . medical approaches are not always the best, with their excessive emphasis on drugs, surgery, and crisis intervention." The book includes information on both biomedical and alternative approaches to health care.

Each of these criticisms of mainstream medicine—excessive cost, skewed access, inadequate current health care organizations, and lack of medical effectiveness—has its own history, proponents, strengths, and weaknesses. Yet increasingly they are presented as a coherent whole, reinforcing and deepening each other. Demonstrations that a particular treatment is not very efficacious are strengthened if the treatment is also costly. Organizational arrangements that lead to reductions in desired treatments are all the worse if the reductions are justified by the need for raising corporate profits, or the treatments are allocated such that those most in need are least likely to receive them.

Criticisms of medicine and the organization of health care services are widespread across the political spectrum, and these views have taken on a quality of enhanced legitimacy. The coming together of these strands of critical thinking was epitomized in the findings and proposals of President Clinton's Health Care Commission. The commission's final report premised each of its proposals on the acceptance of the criticisms we've just described. The politicians who rejected, and eventually scuttled, the report's conclusions did so not on the basis of a rejection of its premises about the costliness, inefficiencies, or ineffectiveness of medicine. Rather, their opposing views were based upon belief that more governmental intervention would make things worse and/or that a greater role by market driven economic forces, not government mandates, could rectify the situation. Extensive criticism of medicine as an institution in American society is now commonly articulated at high levels of the government, the academy, *and* the corporate sector of the economy.

The Synergy of Complaint: Birth of a Grievance

A time like our own, when intensive criticism of medicine has become widespread, offers the potential for even more fundamental critiques and proposals for change. It has not been lost on observers or practitioners that the longstanding critiques of Western medicine as mechanistic, reductionist, and technologically biased can be joined with the recent criticisms of high cost, limited access, inefficiency, and therapeutic ineffectiveness. Taken together, the impact of both sets of criticisms is more than the sum of the parts. If medicine is not only too costly, inaccessible, and ineffective but also fundamentally wrong in its most basic assumptions about the nature of illness and healing, significant improvement can only come through a major change in how we think about health and healing. The problems are so great that a solution will require the emergence of what some have termed a new "paradigm."

The relatively common use of the terms "paradigm" and "paradigm shift" is traceable to Thomas Kuhn's *The Structure of Scientific Revolutions.* Kuhn used examples from physics to rebut the idea that scientific change came about through the consistent and gradual accretion of knowledge among experts. Rather, Kuhn asserted, change was generated in bursts—as the accumulation of facts or insights that disproved existing doctrines took hold among researchers who were outside the scientific mainstream. These outsiders focused their thoughts and theories on the inevitable gaps or lapses in what the dominant perspective could explain. A new paradigm was "revolutionary" in Kuhn's view because it aggressively pointed out the deficiencies of the old ways of seeing, and because it offered a new way of understanding in place of the old. The extent to which the new paradigm helped people understand something heretofore incomprehensible would determine its success. Kuhn himself was surprised, and eventually somewhat aghast, at the way his descriptions of changes in physics became used to describe changes (or proposed changes) in many arenas of intellectual and social life. It was far from clear to Kuhn that something as vast as "medicine" was very much like the small world of theoretical physics. Still, both advocates and observers of alternative medicine use Kuhn's terminology in describing the "paradigm shift" to a new "medical model." For example, Deepak Chopra writes, "Each assumption of the old paradigm can be replaced with a more complete and expanded version of the truth." In his call for "a new medical model," Kenneth Pelletier asserts:

> Medicine, based upon Newtonian physics, has adhered for some time to one mode of scientific inquiry with inherent assets and often-unacknowledged limitations. . . . Holistic approaches to health parallel the insights of quantum physics in that both supplant the Newtonian reductionist view of the world with the quantum perspective of a dynamic universe. From this new paradigm derive the philosophical and scientific roots for the practice of holistic medicine.

In using this language, these and many other alternative practitioners "suggest that a holistic approach to health care is so original that it qualifies as a paradigm shift, that is, an entirely new way of characterizing and approaching the problems of a given discipline."

Whether or not alternative medicine does offer a truly new paradigm is open to question. In part the answer lies in specifying whether those who advocate an "alternative medicine" hold a common set of conceptual understandings. This is the subject of the next chapter. But, the answer depends as well on the ability of the new paradigm to successfully respond to the gaps or failures of the dominant biomedical paradigm. An "alternative" paradigm requires something to which it is an alternative. In this respect it differs from a paradigm that claims to be "holistic," "complementary," or "integrative." It is the very ability to point out, emphasize, and respond to the various failures of something else that energizes and gives a raison d'etre to anything that is self-consciously "alternative."

Alternative medicine *does* represent a new paradigm in that it provides a new framing of ideas about illness and the health care system. Situations and circumstances that were previously seen as uncomfortable or unfortunate now are conceptualized as being wrong or unjust. For example, the standard biomedical approaches for treatment of chronic illness and suffering are not just perceived as inadequate but as grievously and unacceptably limited. Alternative medicine offers the sense that the current situation is riddled with contradictions and that something else, something better, is possible. The future of alternative medicine hinges on its ability to prove that such an approach to health and illness does exist. But, the opportunity for alternative medicine to make its case at this point in history derives from the extent, depth, and acceptance of the notion that existing forms of conventional medicine have come to place an unreasonable burden upon society and hinder our ability to respond to illness.

The phenomena described in the following pages are called by many names: holistic medicine, mind-body medicine, East-West medicine, complementary medicine, integrative medicine, and more. The advocates of each term are cogent in offering reasons for why their particular choice best encapsulates the underlying principles of the techniques they use. Often, these advocates disdain the term "alternative medicine" because of its residual character. Alternative medicine is what conventional medicine is not. From a purely clinical perspective this reasoning may be sound, if not persuasive. But the phrase "alternative medicine" best captures the role and meaning of these techniques and approaches to healing in relation to the larger society.

3 The Core of Alternative Medicine

Age-Old Wisdom Made New

Attending an alternative medicine conference, scanning the titles shelved under the heading of alternative medicine in a "megastore," or "surfing the net" for sites related to alternative medicine can be both an overwhelming and a puzzling experience. The sheer volume of what is readily available, no less its vague boundaries and overlapping categories, are, at best, confusing. Beyond the rhetorical titles of some of the most popular works (*Total Health; Everyday Miracles; Ageless Body, Timeless Mind*), the wide range of approaches, techniques, and philosophies encompassed is striking. There are specific healing techniques such as aromatherapy, flower remedies, massage, guided imagery, and acupuncture. Then there are entire systems of medicine: Traditional Chinese Medicine (TCM), Ayurvedic medicine, naturopathy, homeopathy, and mind-body medicine, among others. And there are other things that would seem to be more than a specific technique but less than a fully developed system of medicine, such as qigong, yoga, and herbal medicine. Finally, there are the so-called "New Age" phenomena like crystal healing and psychic healing, which defy simple classification.

What, if anything, do these have in common? One thing they have in common is that they have typically *not* been taught about in American medical schools, *not* been utilized by most physicians and hospitals, and *not* reimbursed for by most in-

40

surance plans. A definition of alternative medicine based upon what it *is not* is therefore both accurate and convenient. It avoids the need to become embroiled in conceptual questions about the assumptions that underlie words like "health," "illness," and "healing." Not surprisingly, it is this straightforward empirical approach to defining alternative medicine that is used by the federal government and mainstream medicine. The Office of Alternative Medicine at the National Institutes of Health defines alternative medicine as "an unrelated group of nonorthodox therapeutic practices, often with explanatory systems that do not follow conventional biomedical explanations." In the study conducted by Daniel Eisenberg and his colleagues that appeared in the prestigious *New England Journal of Medicine* and is the most frequently cited academic report on the subject, alternative medicine was defined as "medical interventions not taught widely at U.S. medical schools or generally available at U.S. hospitals."

Historically, there has been no alternative medicine, but rather many alternative medicines, each separate in its own mind. Practitioners of these alternative modes of care have often viewed each other competitively and acted accordingly, practicing in isolation from one another. Until recently, the various forms of alternative medicine had only been linked negatively by more conventional groups as health fraud or quackery. Organizations like the American Medical Association have been quite willing to describe the approaches now called "alternative medicine" as united by their ignorance, foolishness, and irrationality.

But to define alternative medicine only by what it *is not* avoids important questions about its fundamental nature as well as that of mainstream medicine. The power, prestige, and authority, not to mention financial rewards, accrued by mainstream medicine have typically been justified by its practitioners as emerging from the application of scientific rationality to medical practice. Whatever is taught in medical school, or practiced on patients, is assumed by the general public to have some scientific basis. If a specific technique can become "mainstream" simply by its inclusion in a mainstream institution such as a medical school, what role does that leave for scientific rationality as an arbiter? Accepting an exclusively residual definition of alternative medicine may be pragmatically useful, but it is not very helpful in understanding the larger questions about the differences between mainstream and alternative medicine. More importantly, for our purposes, accepting a residual definition alone makes it difficult to understand the growing power and popularity of those techniques and approaches that comprise alternative medicine. If there are underlying themes within this cacophony of concepts, approaches, and techniques, then starting with the assumption that they do not exist will make them harder to find.

There is no shortage of alternative medical practitioners who emphatically state that there *are* underlying commonalities to the wide range of alternative techniques. A number of earlier academic observers have been able to extract a coherent set of common themes from their studies of the topic. However, to specify a conceptually cohesive set of common elements does not necessarily indicate that they are apparent in the everyday practice of alternative medicine. Thus, in laying out the essential core beliefs within alternative medicine (and they are not radically different from those set out by others), my goal will be to show how they pervade the diverse range of alternative techniques and approaches.

In order to assess whether or not a cohesive set of core beliefs underlies alternative medicine, we should keep in mind a sense of perspective about the real world. A core set of beliefs in the practice of alternative medicine will likely be no more sharply defined and operational than are core beliefs in the practice of mainstream medicine. In the latter we find brain surgery, psychopharmacology, medical genetics, and psychoanalysis coexisting along with scores of other specialties. Such variety doesn't preclude a common set of beliefs in biomedicine. Rather, it indicates that not every practitioner or specialty relates to these beliefs in the same way, or to the same degree. This is likely to be true in alternative medicine as well.

Some observers of alternative medicine have seen only a hodgepodge of practices and points of view, and scoff at the notion that the phrases "alternative medicine" or "holistic medicine" characterize a uniform set of beliefs. As one such researcher commented, "No uniform set of holistic therapies can be identified . . . so much diversity exists among the proponents of holism that it can scarcely be considered a single movement." But, a far larger group of commentators, both favorably and unfavorably inclined toward alternative medicine, have discerned an underlying set of core beliefs or assumptions.

Although most observers agree on the existence of a core set of assumptions, there is little consensus on what they are or how many there are. For example, James Gordon, a sympathetic physician writing in 1980, described seventeen distinct elements of what he called "the paradigm of holistic medicine." Almost a decade later, two social scientists, Kristine Alster and June Lowenberg, independently specified twelve core elements operating as "statements and slogans" and "parameters of the new model of holistic medicine" but agreed with the items on each other's list only half the time. More recently, Robert Buckman and Karl Sabbagh found eight "philosophical attractions" common to the work and beliefs of alternative healers, and Bonnie Blair O'Connor found nine "concepts common to many vernacular health belief systems" in her study of alternative medicine. Yet again, however, the lists are in agreement on few of the terms.

This initial appearance of inconsistency is somewhat misleading. A closer reading of these works, and many others, soon reveals that they use a wide array of dissimilar phrases and terms to express a relatively small number of commonly held ideas. A few central themes appear over and over, sometimes with varying emphasis, with elements combined in some schema while distinct in others. Those who have studied this phenomenon do not differ over whether a core set of beliefs exists, or even what these beliefs are. Rather, their differences of opinion revolve around to what extent these core beliefs are actually manifest in alternative medicine as it is practiced in the real world. The relationship between theory and practice is what needs to be ascertained.

In my view, there are six significant points that distinguish alternative medicine from the medical mainstream: a belief in holism; an emphasis on the integration of body, mind, and spirit; a view of health as a positive state on a continuum with illness; a belief that the body is suffused by the flow of energy; a belief in vitalism; and a distinctive view of the healing process.

Holism

Holism is the belief that entities are greater than the sum of their parts. The belief that individuals must be seen in the totality of their lives permeates alternative medicine. Signs or symptoms are not isolated phenomena to be treated. Rather, the entire physical, emotional, spiritual, and social makeup of the person must be considered. The centrality of this belief to most modes of alternative practice is so pronounced that many people prefer to use the term "holistic medicine." Because holism directly contradicts the beliefs in dualism and reductionism that are central to biomedicine, it is holism, most fundamentally, that separates alternative medicine from the premises of the conventional biomedical model. Holism has two fundamental implications for a system of healing. The first, and most frequently described, is the belief in the interpenetration of mind, body, spirit, and the larger environment. Because this tenet is so crucial, it is discussed at length below. However, holism has an even more fundamental implication as well: the uniqueness of the individual.

Holism rejects any separation of the mental and physical realms of life and requires that each individual be seen in terms of his or her uniqueness. In this regard alternative medicine is distinguished from mainstream practice by a matter of degree. Holism is a theme in conventional medical practice, but a relatively minor one. Most mainstream practitioners would concur that individuals are each one of a kind, defined by their own genetic inheritance, personal history, and social position. Nevertheless, in most situations, acknowledging this individuality would have relatively little to do with which specific therapy was offered for a particular set of symptoms, or with the basic understanding of the pathologic processes behind a particular disease. For alternative practitioners, treatment and pathology are often as unique as the person seeking assistance. As Gordon has written, "Each person will require a different approach—different forms of exercise, a different diet, a different pharmacological treatment, and different kinds of psychotherapeutic interventions. One asthmatic adolescent may best be treated in a group that runs several miles a day. Another may be seen in the context of a systems-oriented family therapy. The first may work out her anger and improve her vital capacity through daily running. The second may diminish her anxieties and increase self-confidence through biofeedback techniques."

In practice, this emphasis on the uniqueness of the individual permeates alternative medicine, and for many clients is a source of great comfort. For example, homeopathy, a system of treating symptoms with minute doses of substances ("remedies") that in greater amounts would bring on the symptom, offers an extensive and highly personalized diagnostic encounter with the homeopath. According to homeopath Harris Coulter, "Homeopathy holds that the key to the 'wholeness' of the patient, and of the remedy, is found in their peculiarities or idiosyncrasies—in other words in the factors that distinguish *this* patient and *this* remedy from other patients and other remedies that are similar but not the same as *this* one." In its essence, this view calls the entire biomedical classification of disease into question. Homeopaths and other alternative healers emphasize the immense diversity in symptoms reported by individuals suffering from the same condition or disease: arthritis, gastrointestinal distress, PMS, asthma, etc. They ask why the malady is taking the specific form it has in a particular individual.

The biomedical model accepts symptomatic variation (and indeed even documents it) but justifies the clumping together of symptoms on the basis of an underlying physiopathology. Increasingly, alternative modes of care accept this view but raise questions about what it means. Homeopathy is not opposed to acknowledging that arthritis is usually initiated by a chemically induced inflammation. It asks, Why were these chemicals released? Biomedicine answers by citing a problem in the immune system. But, what caused the immune system to malfunction? Homeopathy says the answer will be different for each individual, as it will for the root cause of high blood pressure or any other condition. Linda Johnston, a well-known homeopath, writes, "Modern medicine doesn't bother speculating about the unknown initiating cause of symptoms. . . . Doctors usually want to know just enough to enable them to eliminate the symptoms. . . . These efforts seem beneficial to the patient, however, the disease causing the symptoms has not been cured, it has only been blocked . . . similar to putting a dam across a river."

Each of the major systems within alternative medicine holds beliefs that are almost identical to those of homeopathy about the importance of individuality in assessing and treating illness. Ayurvedic medicine is a traditional Indian system of healing that uses diet, exercise, meditation, massage, herbs, light, and breathing techniques to treat illness by restoring inner harmony of body, mind and spirit. The best known practitioner of Ayurveda in the United States is Deepak Chopra, who states that "an Ayurvedic physician is more interested in the patient he sees before him than in his disease. He recognizes that what makes up the person is experience—sorrows, joys, fleeting seconds of trauma, long hours of nothing special at all. The minutes of life silently accumulate, and like grains of sand deposited by a river, the minutes can eventually pile up into a hidden formation that crops above the surface as disease."

Traditional Chinese Medicine (TCM) is a three thousand-year-old system that combines acupuncture, diet, massage, herbs, and other treatments to enhance and restore health. The techniques that comprise TCM all explicitly reject treating specific symptoms. Rather, they view problems as reflecting the character of the individual, as expressed through combinations of "yin" and "yang," complementary interpenetrating forces that are reflected in bodily functions and organs and exert their energy through twelve bodily meridians.

Naturopathy is a healing system that emerged from the European tradition of herbalism and spa cures, as shaped by the American experience of the Kellogg brothers and their Battle Creek–based sanitarium and health food business. Today its practitioners, licensed in a number of states, utilize a melange of techniques including herbal medicine, hydrotherapy, physical manipulation, homeopathy, and many others. Despite its eclectic nature and the absence of an overarching theoretical system, there is explicit consensus about the necessity of focusing on the person, not on symptoms or disease. This conceptualization is essentially identical to that of TCM.

Holism is the most commonly held premise among all alternative medical systems. It is also a view that resonates strongly with fundamental values in American culture regarding the importance and uniqueness of the individual. In this affinity with a core American value, holism offers a connection to the nation's history and collective psyche. This linkage gives alternative medicine the opportunity to present itself as the embodiment of the most legitimate of the culture's goals: allowing individuals to freely assert their individuality.

The Interpenetration of Mind, Body, and Spirit

Most mainstream physicians would agree that the body and mind are intimately related, and that changes in one are often related to changes in the other. What is distinctive about alternative medicine is, again, the extent and degree of emphasis put on this relationship, along with the common inclusion of "spirit" as a separate dimension. This fundamental premise affects almost every aspect of alternative treatment.

The intimate interconnection of body and mind is a basic assumption of nearly every non-Western system of medicine. Over the past several decades, aspects of these systems have increasingly found support from two distinct strains of Western science. Social psychologists and social epidemiologists have consistently reported that people who are chronically unhappy, depressed, lonely, and stressed are more likely to suffer from just about every type of physical disorder. Simultaneously, the laboratory-based field of psychoneuroimmunology (PNI) has blossomed by convincingly demonstrating that emotional states can alter chemicals in the body. Neuropeptides and their receptors throughout the body have come to be seen as the biochemical dimension of emotion. At first it was believed that these chemicals, of which the pleasure producing endorphins are the best known, were confined to the brain. But now it has been established that they operate throughout the body, especially on the endocrine and immune systems—the very parts of the organism that fight disease. The link between emotions and the body that alternative medical systems had long described can now be specified in a Western scientific vocabulary. The means by which the emotionally "created" neuropeptide enters a cell is identical to the way a virus enters the same cell.

PNI has made the observations of social scientists seem like confirmations of what laboratory experiments would predict. Equally as important have been the findings that people can, to some significant degree, control the processes described by

PNI. Despite the rapid accumulation of such findings, PNI and related scientific advances have had relatively little impact on the practice of conventional medicine. Even when mainstream physicians accept the findings, they are unsure of how to utilize them in their daily work or are unable to do so. The rise of "managed care," where access to the doctor and the amount of time per visit are more strictly rationed, has heightened the difficulty of using these results in most conventional medical settings.

These findings, which support the interpenetration of body and mind, have had a major impact on the field of alternative medicine *beyond* merely substantiating one of its core beliefs. Because the interpenetration of body and mind is inextricably intertwined with many other essential elements of the alternative worldview, these results have validated and energized the full range of alternative core beliefs. Thus, when *JAMA* reports that emotions like sadness and frustration reduce the supply of blood to the heart sufficiently to double or triple the risk of ischemia, the idea of mind-body interpenetration is supported. But, as individuals vary so greatly in what frustrates them and how they react to frustration, the importance of holism is validated as well.

Simply knowing that a biological pathway may connect the mind and body provides little guidance on exactly how to utilize such a link to help someone else who is ill. For the most part, straightforward willfulness seems ineffective. Thus, someone with hypertension may know the mind can lower or raise blood pressure, but simply "telling" your body that you truly want to reduce your blood pressure will do nothing. The power of the mind over the body appears to operate indirectly. Individuals must be able to conceptualize and truly believe in the process in a way that is meaningful and acceptable to them. What will work for one person will not necessarily work for the next, because some conceptualizations of the process may not be compatible with the beliefs and experiences of certain people. Andrew Weil illustrates this point by describing the huge number of different techniques that have been used to rid people's bodies of warts, ranging from handling some kind of animal to being touched by a wart healer. All the cures he cites operate via suggestion, the potential dominance of the mind over the body. Yet individuals vary tremendously in which suggestions work for them. Thus, understanding that the mind has the ability to cure a wart under certain conditions, which will vary from person to person, tends to support the idea that each person actualizes this potential in a unique way.

The belief in the interpenetration of body, mind, and spirit is at the heart of all the healing systems that comprise alternative medicine. TCM and its constituent techniques, such as acupuncture and herbs, all hold that "the unseen and the seen, psyche and soma are mutually valid and co-generative." Similar views are found in Ayurvedic medicine and in yoga. The term "yoga" means union, and its basic principle is the unity of body and mind. The systematic presentation of yoga in its eight "limbs" and its postures, breathing exercises, and meditation are all explicitly directed toward bringing mind, body, and spirit into harmony for the mutual goals of physical vitality, mental clarity, and spiritual awareness.

Many of the alternative techniques commonly used for healing in the United States are derived from TCM and Ayurvedic medicine: meditation, biofeedback, guided imagery, neurolinguistic therapy, etc. Although they are often presented or "packaged" without their roots in these older and broader systems of healing and spirituality, they always are most explicit about the interplay of mind and body. "Transcendental Meditation" (which has been commodified to the extent that the term itself is trademarked) is an easily learned form of meditation based in the Vedic tradition of Indian spirituality. Since the late 1950s, at least four million people have taken an introductory course on its practice. The course stresses the technique's ability to bring about physiological changes, such as reduction in blood pressure, improvement in immune functioning, and mental calmness. In many settings where meditation is taught and practiced, the mind-body linkage is the initial focus of the practice. However, as most advocates and observers have noted, the more a person meditates, the more he or she moves toward the goal of spiritual growth and enlightenment. As the interpenetration of body and mind are more fully accepted or recognized by the individual, a belief in vitalism and the role of the spirit is fostered.

Biofeedback and guided imagery are both specific techniques for teaching people how to use their minds to control their internal physical states. In biofeedback, participants are given continuous information from electronic devices that measure physiological variables. Then they are encouraged to explore precisely which mental states, thoughts, etc., will influence their internal state. As the participants gain skill, they can invoke the beneficial states at will, without the feedback from the electronic devices. Guided imagery encourages the users to delve into their own personal history or fantasies to conjure up images that enable them to control their internal states. Proponents of each technique cite evidence showing the technique is effective for treating a wide range of stress-related disorders such as migraines, tension headaches, hypertension, insomnia, sinusitis, and tachycardia, along with many other problems such as neurological disorders, cardiac irregularities, epilepsy, and fecal incontinence. Advocates of guided imagery also claim benefit for "fighting" many forms of cancer, as well as AIDS. The roots of guided imagery derive from both TCM and Ayurvedic medicine. Biofeedback emerged from academic research in psychophysiology and the work of cognitive psychologists attempting to understand the relation of thought, perception, emotion, and the body. In each instance, the development of the technique was premised upon the assumption of the interpenetration of body and mind.

Since biofeedback, meditation, and guided imagery have a

common—if not always acknowledged—set of roots in traditional healing systems, it is not surprising that they stress body-mind interaction. But most other alternative techniques emphasize mind-body interactions as well. For example, there is an array of healing techniques that rely on body movement and touching, such as shiatsu massage, Rolfing, the Alexander Technique, Feldenkrais, chiropractic, Reichian therapy, and bioenergetics. Despite the fact that each primarily involves physical manipulation of the body, the manipulation is given meaning by being placed within the context of mind-body interaction, along with the other basic premises of alternative thought.

In some cases the relationship of body and mind is viewed as nonspecific, affecting one's overall health. Examples include the overall enhancement of emotions and improved clarity of thought that are claimed as benefits of massage, the improved physical alignment of the body from Rolfing, and the lengthening of the spine to allow proper neck alignment in the Alexander Technique. Other therapeutic modalities manipulate a specific body part to affect a particular aspect of the individual's mental health. For example, Feldenkrais maintains that specific movements and postures create a person's "self image," and that gradually altering how individuals position themselves in physical space can fundamentally influence their personal growth. A follower of Rolfing created Hellerwork specifically to incorporate the emotional aspect into the physical manipulations developed by Ida Rolf. In its focus on emotional and physical release, Hellerwork is similar to bioenergetics, the technique developed by Alexander Lowen, a Reichian psychiatrist. Reich, a student of Freud, believed that posture and breathing reflected whatever psychic traumas had been inflicted upon people early in their lives. He devised verbal and physical mechanisms to release the mental trauma held in physical form by the individual. Ida Rolf built her theories on his work. In many respects Reich's ideas are almost identical to the theories underlying TCM, which are reflected in shiatsu massage, acupressure, and many other techniques. Mind-body interaction is at the root of all of them.

The best known and most widely used of the alternative physical manipulation techniques is chiropractic. Chiropractic was founded in the late 1800s by Daniel David Palmer, who believed all people had "innate intelligence" that, if unimpeded, would create a state of perfect health in the body. As currently practiced, chiropractic's views about the interplay of body, mind, and spirit vary greatly. Yet as originally put forth by Palmer, its fundamental principle was "the acknowledgement that life is an expression of a divine or metaphysical reality." Palmer saw his contribution as the specification of exactly how this divine spirit, "the Innate," operated on a physical level in the body. He believed the spirit entered through the brain, then traveled via the nerves throughout the body. It was for this reason that the alignment of the vertebrae was key to ensuring good health. For Palmer, the physical, moral, and spiritual elements of life and healing were all part of "a tightly woven core." The founder's son, B. J. Palmer, who is responsible for much of chiropractic's growth as a profession, concurred with his father's beliefs. He renamed "the Innate" as "Universal Intelligence" and claimed this as the scientific name for what other religions called God, Buddha, or Jehovah. Today organized chiropractic has abandoned most explicit mentions of its origins. But, it still maintains that its manipulations work by enhancing the body's own ability to utilize "higher" forces.

The idea that some purely physical intervention fosters the transmission of psychological and/or spiritual forces that bring about healing appears in a number of alternative modes of care besides chiropractic. The use of flower extracts for healing, Bach Flowers being the most widely known system, operates upon the same premises. Edward Bach, an English physician, believed that most illness was psychosomatic in nature. Practicing in the 1930s, he felt that medicine had no real cures for the problems that beset his patients but provided only symptomatic relief. He came to believe that the extracts of thirty-eight wild flowers would profoundly affect the underlying psychological causes of most illness. Choice of a particular remedy was based upon a holistic view of the patient; symptoms were secondary. Histories of herbal medicine are clear that it is fundamentally built on a set of spiritual beliefs concerning nature's ("the great spirit") ability to enter the mind and body through plants. In both TCM and Ayurvedic medicine the use of herbs reflects the systems' broader understandings of the connection between the mind and the body.

The interpenetration of body, mind, and spirit is clearly an essential element common to almost all the belief systems and techniques that make up alternative medicine. As in the case of holism, this belief is sometimes present in conventional medicine. However, the distinction is again one of degree and emphasis. The interpenetration of body, mind, and spirit as a means of healing has also been repeatedly expressed in health and religious movements from William Alcott's Christian Physiology Movement in the 1850s, through Ellen White's Seventh Day Adventism, and Graham's clinics in Battle Creek, Michigan, evangelists like Gordon Lindsey, Oral Roberts and today's charismatic and evangelical churches. Public opinion polls consistently show that the vast majority of the population, regardless of religion or religiosity, accepts the intimate connection between body, mind, and spirit. To the extent that alternative medicine is based upon a similar premise, it is allied with a longstanding view held by most Americans.

Health as a Positive State on a Continuum with Illness

Despite the fact that the nation has been concerned with *health* reform, and many people have *health* insurance and a regular *health* care provider, these things are almost solely concerned with illness, not health. The dominant tendency within biomedicine has been to treat illness or disease. Illness is usually seen as an entity—someone *has* a heart attack or the measles—albeit frequently an entity that has known precursors and sequelae. In conventional "mainstream" medical practice, health is the absence of illness.

For the vast majority of alternative approaches and practitioners, however, health is not merely the absence of diagnosable disease; it is something positive to which individuals aspire and can attain through their efforts. Reducing or eliminating symptoms, preventing future illness, and striving toward a high(er) level of health or wellness are not separate activities. As health and illness are understood as points on a personal continuum, anyone can always be healthier. Preventing future illness, disability, or "dis-ease" receives much greater prominence from alternative providers than it does in mainstream medicine. For many alternative approaches, the term "health" often takes on a transcendent quality. Whatever one's physical or mental state, whether terminally ill or a championship athlete, it is always possible to be healthier. Awareness of the possibilities for change, education about how to actualize these possibilities, and personal growth are all part of being healthy. In this quest energy, optimism, and inner peace are often cited as manifestations of "health."

Whereas mainstream medicine has often treated health as an afterthought and prevention as something to be addressed after the overwhelming tide of disease and symptoms have been dealt with, alternative approaches are much more likely to offer health as their primary goal. The view of health in homeopathy is typical of most alternative systems. Linda Johnston explains: "Defining health in terms of a lack of disease, pain or disability, implies that by eliminating these conditions we will restore health. This is simply not so. That is similar to stating that we are financially secure if we are not in debt. . . . The mere absence of debt compared to all the possibilities there are with an abundance of money is similar to the difference between the absence of disease and experiencing true health."

In *Quantum Healing,* Deepak Chopra states that "Ayurveda

is commonly classified as a system of medicine, but with equal justice you could call it a system for curing delusions, for stripping away the convincing quality of disease and letting a healthier reality take its place." For Chopra revelation, bliss, and enlightenment are the essence of health. It is by attaining these states, and by being in a state of transcendence, that the healing techniques of Ayurveda can be utilized. Being healthy is a prerequisite to alleviating disease, rather than the outcome or evidence of a cure. Indeed, being healthy removes an "invisible barrier" and enables the body to age more slowly without "trying." In support of this idea, Chopra cites a study which found that the typical sixty-year-old who has meditated for at least five years will have the physiology of a forty-eight-year-old.

TCM maintains similar notions of health as a positive state on a continuum with illness. TCM is "more preventive in nature than conventional medicine, and views the practice of waiting to treat a disease until the symptoms are full blown as being similar to digging a well after one has become thirsty." The human body is seen as a reflection of the natural world, and the health of an individual is analogous to a state of ecological balance in nature. The forces of yin and yang describe the interdependence of fluctuating opposites. Creating a balance between them is synonymous with health. The guiding premise of TCM is that "the superior physician cures before the illness is manifested. The inferior physician can only treat the illness he was unable to prevent." Acupuncture, perhaps the best known aspect of TCM in the West, has an understanding of health that is identical to the larger system of TCM.

Chiropractic's "adjustments" or manipulations of the spine and joints are intended to allow the "innate intelligence" of the body to cure disorders that arise from systemic blockages, or "subluxations." Health is the positive state of being free from these blockages. In each of the major alternative healing systems, health is the idea of a positive state, not simply the removal of symptoms or pathology.

The same view of health extends to the practice of most alternative techniques that are not, by themselves, complete systems of healing. An example is biofeedback, whose goal is to produce a state of health far beyond the alleviation of symptoms. Once a patient's blood pressure and respiration improve, the goal of biofeedback becomes health, or perfect functioning. This is expressed by some exponents as "a drugless high" similar to that experienced by yogis. Guided imagery is similar to biofeedback, in that although many people initially use it for the alleviation of a specific problem, it intentionally moves the participant toward broader goals such as insight, creativity, and a general state of well being.

Qigong and yoga, which both originated in non-Western societies, conceive of health in ways that are strikingly similar to the principles behind biofeedback and guided imagery, which were developed in the West. Qigong, an ancient Chinese exercise regimen incorporating body movement, meditation, and control of respiration is, by one estimate, practiced daily by over two hundred million people in China. The qigong tradition emphasizes the importance of teaching the patient how to remain well. In China, qigong is the nucleus of a national self-care system of health maintenance and personal development. According to practitioners, "qigong cultivates inner strength, calms the mind, and restores the body to its natural state of health." The traditional practice of yoga offers an even more fully developed concept of health organized around eight "limbs," which bring full integration of a person via heightened spiritual awareness and physical purification.

Although many mainstream health care providers might endorse the notion that health is more than simply the absence of symptoms, alternative systems and approaches typically go well beyond this. They consistently support the sense that both disease and wellness are different points on a single continuum that reflects the underlying relationship of the person to the larger world. Being healthy involves constantly striving to improve. The striving itself is a key aspect of being truly healthy, as well as a creator of future health. The experience of working with a practitioner to achieve a greater sense of health, as opposed to passively letting a physician cure you or rid you of symptoms, is a crucial aspect of alternative medicine. The language of many alternative health systems, used to define health and the means of attaining it, may at first seem "foreign" or exotic. But, its meaning often reiterates classic American ideals which assert that everyone, no matter how bad off, can and should better themselves. The tone of alternative medicine is eternally optimistic in its focus on striving and the possibility of achievement. In alternative medicine the nature of the therapeutic encounter, and the specific treatments themselves, all emerge from this fundamental assumption.

Life Suffused by the Flow of Energy

The flow of energy is what ties together the various elements of mind, body, spirit, and environment for most alternative healing systems and techniques. When the flow of energy is blocked, or in some way skewed, illness emerges. Although there may be some general idea about what a "balance" of energy means in the abstract (for example, the balancing of yin and yang in TCM), in real life energy flows from an infinite variety of paths. The causes of illness and the sources of health and healing are unique to each person.

The importance of energy flow is seen most easily in TCM, which posits a basic life force variously called "qi" or "chi" that flows throughout the body. TCM techniques, such as acupuncture, work by keeping the qi flowing so that each of the body's organs can operate efficiently and support the others. Qi's ability to flow properly is crucial because the body's ten basic organs are understood to reflect five aspects of the outside physical world (e.g., the heart and small intestine represent fire, the lungs and large intestine represent metal). TCM teaches that understanding how the forces of the natural world remain in balance helps bring harmony to the internal world of the individual: "The human body is viewed as an ecosystem . . . each person has a unique terrain to be mapped, a resilient yet sensitive ecology to be maintained." It is especially important to balance each pair of organs that reflect the same element in the physical world, as one is the "yin" organ and the other the "yang."

The qi energy can be transmitted from the environment or another person, or enhanced within oneself. The healer's own qi can enter the patient. In the widely viewed TV series "Healing and the Mind," Bill Moyers, the host, asked David Eisenberg, an American physician who studied TCM in China: "When the doctor does acupuncture, does he use his own chi?" Eisenberg replied, "Yes, I have to use my chi to stick the needle in. I also spin the needle, which requires a lot of skill. If I do it with the emission of my chi, the patient will have an intense feeling."

Ayurvedic medicine holds similar ideas to TCM with regard to the role of energy. According to the principles of Ayurveda, the body is like a river, defined by its ever changing flow. Chopra has criticized biomedicine for its disregard of this flow: "The first thing killed in the laboratory is the delicate web of intelligence that binds the body together." As in TCM, Ayurveda asserts that the ultimate source of health lies in accepting the apparently contradictory notion that individuality is illusory. It is only a reflection of the "flow" of the larger universe: "Disease is the result of a disruption of the spontaneous flow of nature's intelligence within our physiology." The vast majority of the many forms of meditation are built upon the fundamental tenets of either Ayurvedic medicine or TCM. According to one practitioner, "From the meditative perspective . . . health was not some kind of static thing that you grab and run with to the goal line. Health is a dynamic energy flow that changes over a lifetime. In fact, health and illness often coexist together."

Most other major alternative healing systems, such as homeopathy and chiropractic, assign a similar role to energy. In homeopathy, symptoms of illness occur when life is out of balance. The usual causes of illness, such as a virus, will have limited impact upon someone whose body, mind, and emotions are in balance. Therefore, if the natural homeostatic state is disrupted, the balance must be restored. The "defense mechanisms" of the body are thought to do much of the restorative work by themselves. Thus, homeopathic remedies are prescribed not to remove symptoms, but to stimulate the body's own healing powers to maintain a balance between defense and disease. These powers involve the interactions of body, mind, and emotion via the flow of energy among them. Chiropractic's theory of "Universal Intelligence" and reliance on physical manipulation to remove blockages that otherwise would result in dysfunction is also based on a belief in the centrality of energy flow.

Many other less systematic and less well-known alternative techniques also rely heavily upon notions of balancing or maintaining energy flow through the body. Applied kinesiology—a method of restoring postural balance, improving range of motion, and enhancing muscle functioning—is a good example, as are various forms of therapeutic massage. Each operates on the premise that problems such as poor circulation, lymphatic damage, glandular dysfunction, and immune system disorders can be remedied by releasing muscular blockages that restrict energy flow within the body. A wide array of approaches, often grouped together under the name of "energy medicine," use various electrical devices to both diagnose and measure the body's imbalances, as well as restore them. One compendium of alternative techniques estimates that between eighty-five thousand and a hundred thousand practitioners currently use such techniques in the United States. The manner by which the various electrical devices (such as the "Dermatron," "electroacupuncture," "Electro-Acuscope,"

"Diapulse," and "Infratonic QGM") initiate cures is frequently described as restoring the body's vibrational balance, which in turn leads to improved energy flow. This is almost identical to the explanation that practitioners who use flower remedies offer to explain why their technique works on myriad physical disorders. Other approaches, such as "neural therapy," consist of injecting chemicals into the body to remove blockages, while others aim to remove chemicals considered to cause blockage due to their toxicity. Examples of the latter are various fasting regimens as well as "chelation therapy," in which ethylene-diaminetetraacetic acid (EDTA) is fed intravenously and then (after supposedly binding with various toxins) flushed from the body.

Alternative medicine's emphasis on the flow of energy as a source of healing is distinctive. Unlike the positive definition of health and the interpenetration of body, mind and spirit, it is hardly used at all in mainstream biomedicine. Views such as Chopra's, that the individual is an illusory representation of a universal energy source, are not likely to be taught in American medical schools anytime soon. Nor, for the most part, are such views deeply rooted in American history or values. Perhaps it is for this reason that many alternative practitioners, like chiropractors, play down these ideas and put forth a more mechanistic emphasis on blockages and balance. Regardless of these efforts to use a more congenial vocabulary, an emphasis on the diffusion of energy through the body as a healing force remains a key element of the alternative worldview.

Vitalism

Vitalism, the belief in a basic "life force" that naturally promotes healing, is another important element in many alternative approaches. This belief in a natural tendency toward healing is not entirely absent in mainstream biomedicine. However, in mainstream medicine, the body's own tendency toward healing is seen as less important than the role that the doctor or the treatment plays in bringing about healing and cure. Alternative "practitioners view themselves as midwives to the body's own resources. . . . Instead of trying to eradicate illness, they may attempt to strengthen the body so it can rid itself of disease."

Vitalism is an explicit component of most alternative medical systems. The power of chi or qi in TCM is a clear example. By allowing qi to flow, the body's natural tendency toward health is enhanced. This is the reason heart rate and blood pressure decrease, sleep improves, and immune functioning and oxygen flow increase.

The primary principle of naturopathy, which combines techniques from many alternative traditions, is to facilitate healing through the power of nature. This includes using nontoxic therapies and enhancing patients' power to heal themselves. As in TCM and Ayurvedic medicine, the goal is to cure the person, not the illness. The principle of vitalism provides the basis for much of the naturopathic goal of removing toxic substances from our diets. Pesticides, synthetic food additives such as Aspartame, MSG, dyes, sulfites, etc., are all rejected by naturopaths both because they can cause illness themselves and because they inhibit the body's own ability to heal itself. From the perspective of naturopathy and many other alternative approaches, the distinction between prevention and cure via proper nutrition is arbitrary. This can be seen in the scores of dietary regimens offered by alternative healers, such as Dean Ornish's widely cited therapy for cardiovascular problems, which makes minimal distinction between prevention and treatment.

Herbal medicine is the use of natural substances found in plants to cure illness by enhancing the body's own power. Mainstream medicine acknowledges that plants may have therapeutic power. The World Health Organization Bulletin notes that about a quarter of all contemporary prescription drugs derive originally from plants, and that three-quarters of these medicines are used to treat the same problems for which the plants were traditionally used. But herbalism is more than the treatment of symptoms with plants. In both TCM and Ayurvedic medicine, the use of specific plants corresponds to the overarching vitalistic theories of health. In TCM the five basic elements (metal, earth, fire, water, and wood) are each associated with a specific taste, such as bitterness or sweetness. Treatment is not only based upon the empirical effect of these herbs. Rather, it takes into account the five basic elements and the organs they represent, along with the patient's personality and physical symptoms. In Ayurveda there are also five basic elements. These combine to form three basic body humors (vata, pitta, kapha) that must be kept in balance. In both TCM and Ayurveda, herbs—also classified by taste—are used to restore the balance of the life force.

While much of the herbal medicine currently practiced in the United States is largely symptom based, naturopathy and many other alternative approaches such as flower remedies and aromatherapy use plants and their essences in a manner much more similar to the traditional healing systems. Vitalist tendencies can also be present in other approaches that posit some sort of fundamental health enhancing power, such as the Universal Intelligence found in chiropractic.

The Healing Process

A final feature common to most alternative approaches is their distinctive view of the healing process, and the role of the healer. In many respects, it is this characteristic that most consistently differentiates alternative from mainstream care. Most mainstream physicians reconfigure a patient's illnesses into "diseases" through the theoretical lens of technical scientific medicine. While biomedicine makes healing synonymous with the removal of symptoms, it does not typically address the other realities such as suffering or, most importantly, the meaning of illness for the patient. Yet, the latter is crucial when dealing with chronic illnesses, which comprise an ever increasing proportion of the disease burden in the United States.

For most alternative approaches, healing is a cooperative process. The healer is a partner or a guide, not an omnipotent, distant authority figure. Norman Cousins, in his "Anatomy of an Illness (As Perceived by the Patient)," captured this dimension when he described his battle with ankylosing spondylitis, a severe systemic collagen illness. The most optimistic assessment for a cure his own physician could give him was one in five hundred; most of the specialists said the chances were zero. But, atypically, this same doctor was fully supportive of Cousins's plans to harness the power of positive emotions, which included systematically viewing old television situation comedy shows to induce laughter. Looking back after twelve years of relief from most of his symptoms, Cousins stated that the "principal contribution made by my doctor to the taming, and possibly the conquest, of my illness was that he encouraged me to believe I was a respected partner with him in the total undertaking."

The most well known aspect of the alternative view of healing is its emphasis on the individual "taking responsibility" for his or her own healing. This goes beyond the increasingly well accepted notion of "taking responsibility for one's health," which commonly refers to avoiding cigarettes, eating properly, exercising regularly, etc., to prevent the onset of illness and maintain a state of "high-level wellness." Rather, it is the belief that a cure always entails commitment on the part of the individual. Curing is an active, not a passive, process. This view does not necessarily mean that the individual is primarily responsible for being sick in the first place, although some do hold to this view of illness as destiny or "karma." It usually means that however the illness has come about, a cure can only come if the person accepts the reality of the illness, and the responsibility for dealing with it. The individual always has the potential to move or stretch the limits of what is possible.

To not accept this potential minimizes, if not eliminates, the chances of cure. The healer and patient are partners. But a partnership is bound to fail if one party is pulling in one direction, the other partner in the other.

Some alternative approaches are explicit about the various ways by which taking responsibility can assist the healing process. They claim it leads to fewer feelings of depression and hopelessness and to enhanced immune functioning, and they point out the power of the placebo effect, etc. Others are less explicit about precisely why or how enhanced responsibility is efficacious but are equally adamant that it is necessary. For example, the texts for practitioners of biofeedback, guided imagery, and various forms of meditation all stress the importance of client motivation and positive expectations. Without this context of mutual positive expectations, which are largely the responsibility of the client, the intervention will likely be of little benefit. Therefore, practitioners are advised to devote much effort to finding those clients who already accept the notion of personal responsibility for health, or those who can be motivated to adopt it.

Alternative healing methods often lead patients away from seeing their illness as "the enemy" to be conquered by stronger medicine, a surgical invasion, or a radioactive attack. The alternative view is of illness as a message, whose meaning must be understood in personal terms before one can respond. Systems like homeopathy, TCM, and Ayurvedic medicine set out elaborate topologies, with almost infinite variations, to assist sufferers in finding out what their particular illness and constellation of symptoms mean about their unique balance of body, mind, and spirit interacting within the larger cosmos. Other approaches, such as guided imagery, meditation, or naturopathy, allow individuals more freedom to arrive at their own understanding of the world. Whatever their degree of latitude, central to all of them is the provision of a meaning for illness, what Larry Dossey refers to as "healing words."

Personal responsibility for healing and partnership with a

healer both imply conscious effort. The essence of alternative healing is a changed consciousness about what is possible. What differentiates the many specific forms of alternative medicine is how this change in consciousness is brought about. It is almost always indirect, as opposed to a simple act of will. Telling your immune system to "get stronger" will do little, if any, good. But repeatedly imagining your white blood cells as small ancient warriors, or a SWAT team, depending on which image appeals most to you, may be more successful. Describing her work with the seriously ill, Naomi Remen, one of the co-founders of Commonweal, a well known center of mind-body medicine in Bolinas, California, states, "Imagery is the way the mind and the body talk to each other . . . [and] the visual is only one way in which we imagine. . . . Some of us are visual, some auditory, some kinesthetic. . . . We all do imagery, but in our own way." Indirect alteration of consciousness is common to almost every major alternative medical system or technique.

In alternative medicine, the stance of the doctor or healer departs radically from the role of the typical mainstream physician. Genuine caring and full participation in the experience of healing are extolled as the highest virtues. The detached, objective technician is reviled. Alternative practitioners speak openly and proudly of their recognition that their patients want sincere caring, compassion, and personal involvement. Alternative practitioners recognize that providing care and nurturing is often the most important thing they do and that without it, cure or benefit is much less likely. It isn't only that alternative healers use touch frequently, they use a "caring touch." Larry Dossey, a well-known exponent of alternative medicine, quotes Paracelsus when he writes, "The main reason for healing is love." While stressing that the "main" reason is not the sole reason, he and advocates of many other alternative healing systems affirm that "love, compassion, caring, and empathy catalyze healing events." Dean Ornish achieved prominence for his views on how dietary change can actually reverse heart disease; he has personally advised Bill Clinton on how to eat healthier. Ornish's latest book, *Love and Survival*, offers what he calls "irrefutable" evidence in support of love's power to prevent illness and forestall death. The truth of this is not something that can be taught in the classroom. It must be experienced, most commonly through one's own healing or personal transformation. Accounts of such experiences are common in the writings of most alternative healers. My own studies of physicians who have come to redefine themselves as "holistic" revealed that they were no different than other primary care physicians in terms of training, board certification, or patient load. What did differentiate them was their personal experiences. Members of the American Holistic Medical Association, and other groups for alternative physicians, were much more likely to have been sick themselves or had spiritual experiences or life crises. The following comment from one alternative physician was typical: "Which influence was most important to me? Having nearly died. It made me face the life I had lived, on my deathbed. That opened the door. I saw I was hungry for life." Another physician told me, "When my ex-husband and I split up, I left the marriage and he was very destroyed. A month or two after we separated, he developed a spontaneous thrombosis of the left subclavian vein, which in a thirty-five-year-old is extremely rare. I knew that he was a very healthy guy, and it was more than coincidental that this came shortly after this very stressful time in his life. I just know that you can make yourself sick, and that has enabled me to see the contribution to people's illnesses." It was subjective, highly personal experiences like these, outside the realm of professional practice, that were decisive in these doctors redefining themselves as alternative physicians. Ornish himself openly describes how his own turn towards alternative medicine emerged from a crisis of doubt, despair, and repeated thoughts of suicide. He turned to a well-known swami, Satchidananda, who led him to yoga, meditation, and vegetarianism—the very approaches that provide the core of what Ornish promotes today.

Writing in the 1950s, the psychiatrist Jerome Frank attempted to place Western medicine in a larger, cross-cultural context to explain *why* it worked, *when* it worked. He concluded that, independent of the therapeutic efficacy of any specific technique, healing was fostered in situations where people had high expectations of success and were motivated to succeed, and where the techniques and healers were able to provide new meanings or ways of symbolizing symptoms. Each of these was more apt to occur in settings where the healers interacted profoundly with those needing healing, and when both parties felt fundamentally enhanced by the process. Although the past five decades have seen each of Frank's major points validated by countless research studies, mainstream biomedicine has tended to view this information as an implicit criticism of its own focus on the potential of scientific medicine to bring about cures. Alternative practitioners either come from systems that acknowledge and require all Frank described, or have eagerly, if implicitly, embraced the power of his conclusions.

Today the doctor's role as a truly caring and compassionate partner in bringing about healing remains an omnipresent, but minor, theme in mainstream practice. Much is written about fostering these qualities through the selection of medical students and the structure of medical training. Conventional practitioners who embody these values are held up as role models. Still, the forces of "managed care" and cost controls have made these qualities more remote than ever in the daily reality of mainstream medicine. A belief in the necessity of a different sort of healing relationship is a major attraction of alternative medicine, and an important element in differentiating it from the medical mainstream.

The Core of Alternative Medicine

The question of whether there is a common set of core beliefs or assumptions that underlie alternative medicine can be answered affirmatively. Despite the variety of words used to describe the components of this core, and the differing emphases the specific components receive, the underlying premises of most alternative healing systems and techniques reveal a very high degree of overlap, cohesion, and synergy. Similarly, the most widely known written accounts of alternative therapies are highly congruous. Most importantly, this set of core assumptions permeates the actual practice of alternative medicine and is not merely an abstract description. This is not to say that all alternative approaches and practitioners equally adhere to, or utilize, these core assumptions. Just as in the relationship of mainstream medical practice to biomedical science, there is a wide range of variation. Still, it is clear that to define alternative medicine primarily as a residual category is inadequate and misleading.

The existence of an analytically distinct core within alternative medicine does not mean that it is recognized as such by all of those who use these techniques, the larger public, mainstream physicians, or public policymakers. Yet, at this point it is reasonable to conclude that this core has the potential to serve as a source of both meaning and identity to those who practice and utilize alternative medicine. These core elements are mutually reinforcing and cohere in a way that enables them to challenge the dominant biomedical understanding of illness, disease, and healing. In this sense the core comprises an ideology, a set of symbols that is capable of reframing the meaning of events in the world.

Taken together, the core elements of alternative medicine present the chance for it to understand and respond to illness differently than mainstream medicine. The core points out the paradoxes, confusions, and inconsistencies in the dominant biomedical model. The core offers concrete examples of events that can take place in real life, despite the claims of the dominant view that say they cannot or dismiss them as random or meaningless. The power of this set of core beliefs lies not in what it can "explain," but in the new sense of possibility it provides. This is the possibility that those who are suffering can achieve health, healing, happiness, and contentment. Simultaneously, it offers a means for avoiding and resisting the dominant biomedical model by exposing its gaps, contradictions, and limitations. At the most general level, the alternative core beliefs offer the hope of transcendence over mortality by directly linking the individual with nature and a purposeful life.

It is worth reiterating that many of the individual components of the alternative core beliefs are compatible with mainstream medicine. A more "holistic" view of health and illness, increased recognition of the interplay between mind and body, and an acknowledgment of the importance of individual differences in the cause and cure of illness are each well accepted notions in contemporary biomedicine. Indeed, advocates of alternative medicine frequently cite developments in areas of established medical research, such as psychoneuroimmunology, as evidence on behalf of their own views. What differentiates alternative medicine is the extent, centrality, and emphasis given to these ideas along with the synergy they take on when viewed, and used, as a whole. Thus, at the most abstract or theoretical level there is the potential for convergence, integration, or assimilation of the mainstream and alternative perspectives.

It is also clear that, taken together, the core beliefs of alternative medicine, regardless of their origins hundreds or thousands of years ago in faraway cultures, provide a current "response" to the well founded, highly rational critiques of biomedicine described in Chapter 2. Mainstream medicine's inadequate consideration of body-mind relationships, neglect of the impact of social relations on health and healing, bureaucratic inefficiencies and impersonality, and extremely high cost each finds its antithesis in the core beliefs of alternative medicine.

The recent growth of alternative medicine comes, in large part, from its contribution to a portrayal of the dominant medical worldview as one in crisis. The core beliefs of alternative medicine offer a way of using ideas already known, but on the periphery of the conventional approach, in a way that challenges the dominant view. The conventional view is presented as having betrayed its long-term and laudable goals through its neglect of things like body-mind interactions. In this sense, the core beliefs of alternative medicine are a "heretical" challenge to an existing orthodoxy.

Equally important to the alternative core's ability to respond to criticisms of mainstream biomedicine is its resonance and congruence with a number of other aspects of contemporary American life. The most important of these is the diminishing sense of expectation about the future that often seems to characterize public sentiment. For the first time in a number of decades, much of the adult population does not envision that their children's income, occupation, housing, and overall well being will be better than their own. Cynicism abounds about the ability of politicians or government programs to improve the lot of most people. The idea of inevitable progress, fueled by scientific discovery, appears increasingly debatable. Views like these have an underlying affinity with the core beliefs of alternative medicine, especially its emphasis on low technology (and perhaps low cost), avoidance of physicians and hospitals, high reliance on one's self, belief in the power of nature and spirituality, and nostalgia for what may appear to have been simpler times.

One of the most potent connections between the values of alternative medicine and the central ethic of American culture lies in the realm of personal responsibility for health. Although this notion is omnipresent in alternative medicine, it has taken on even greater importance in a culture where rugged individualism is often trumpeted as an ideal. The potential for blame and other harsh judgements toward those who are ill is enhanced when approaches, such as Ayurveda or TCM, are imported into American life.

The alternative core is also quite compatible with the values manifest in a number of current influential social movements. Feminism is the most notable of these. The feminist emphasis on "consciousness raising" as a source of personal transformation, or transcendence over existing interpersonal and social relations, is very similar to the alternative view of the role of consciousness in healing. The idea that physical or biological constraints and conditions—such as menopause, PMS, or some forms of depression—are "socially constructed" and thereby alterable via a change in consciousness have much in common with how many alternative approaches understand the origin, meaning, and healing of illness. These same basic ideas that some very personal conditions are socially created, and are amenable to change by "consciousness raising" of one form or another, are pervasive in movements such as those advocating gay liberation, rights for the disabled and chronically ill, triumph over alcohol and drug abuse, various forms of cultural pluralism and, not least, evangelical religious commitment. Most of these groups and movements are also skeptical of the ability of medical professionals, health care institutions, and "objective, value free" science to offer them much benefit. A number of the beliefs at the core of alternative medicine are already familiar and acceptable, if not established as true for many groups in society. The affinities that the core beliefs have with those of other movements, as well as with values like individualism that are longstanding elements in the broader national consciousness, heighten the legitimacy of alternative medicine.

Alternative medicine's core beliefs are also compatible with important societal trends in that they lend themselves to being mass marketed. Mainstream biomedicine, by its very nature, has demanded some degree of "scientific literacy," not to mention access to facilities, procedures, and substances that are, by law, unavailable to most people except through the use of a professional. The situation with regard to alternative medicine is much more fluid. Despite much about alternative medicine being esoteric and requiring the assistance of a healer or professional of some sort, it is clear that alternative medicine is more easily marketed to individuals as something they can "do" themselves. This characteristic means that alternative approaches and techniques have an almost intrinsic appeal to the individuals and institutions adept at mass production and skillful in the marketing of goods and services.

Even more significant is that the high marketability of alternative approaches makes them attractive to the mass media. The economic well-being of mass media enterprises is based upon their ability to attract and hold consumers, and their ability to attract advertisers or sponsors. The core premises of alternative medicine—such as individual responsibility for healing, vitalism that fosters the use of natural substances in healing, and the relatively nontechnical, accessible nature of the procedures—make alternative approaches desirable topics for coverage in the mass media and fertile ground for advertisers.

Alternative medicine does have a core set of beliefs and assumptions. It is, at least potentially, a powerful set of beliefs offering the possibility of health, peace of mind, and transcendence over illness and disability. These core assumptions have reemerged via a synthesis of very old systems of healing and very current advances in science, facilitated by some widely held criticisms of mainstream biomedicine. All of these elements combine to create a new framework that is quite congenial with ideas already held by a significant proportion of the American populace.

4 Medicine and the Spirit

Most of the core assumptions of alternative medicine differ from those of conventional biomedicine by degree and emphasis. Almost all physicians would grant that the mind and body are inseparably linked, and that being healthy is more than merely the absence of symptoms. Alternative and mainstream approaches differ over the extent of these relationships and their relevance to clinical decisions and outcomes. But spirituality, a vital component of most alternative techniques and the overall alternative perspective, is different. The centrality of spirituality to the alternative perspective elicits discomfort, if not hostility, from many conventional practitioners and health care institutions. For some conventional providers, the recognition and acceptance of a spiritual dimension to life, illness, and healing seems to be an affront to the basic premises of scientific medicine.

Alternative medicine largely accepts the conventional "scientific" descriptions of the biological processes and mechanisms that are associated with the onset of disease, or its remission. But alternative medicine also asks, What conditions must be present for the pathology to overpower the body, and what conditions must be present for healing to occur? The answer often includes spiritual along with physical, mental, and/or emotional factors. Today, almost all well-known advocates of alternative medicine stress the importance of spirituality in health and healing. This includes those whose practices have emerged directly from traditional forms of healing, such as Deepak Chopra, as well as those like Larry Dossey, Bernie Siegel, Dean Ornish, and Andrew Weil who identify themselves

74

much more with a scientific point of view grounded in Western rationality.

The prominent role of spiritual or religious beliefs in the histories of almost every major alternative approach is difficult to deny. All of Ayurvedic medicine derives directly from the Vedic tradition in Hinduism, while TCM and the subdisciplines within it, such as acupuncture, are based upon traditional Chinese Taoism. In each of these traditions illness is viewed as a reflection of a life lived in conflict with ultimate principles that, in turn, derive from universal divine law. In some other major alternative perspectives, such as chiropractic and homeopathy, contemporary practitioners sometimes downplay the original spiritual roots of the enterprise. However, their influence continues to be felt. It is striking to what extent the views of D. D. Palmer and other early advocates of chiropractic are almost identical to those of Ayurveda and TCM. Palmer writes: "Chiropractors envisioned man as a microcosm of the universe, with the Innate Intelligence that determined human health to be a manifestation of a larger Universal Intelligence that governed the cosmos." Palmer frequently stated that manipulations of chiropractors that unblocked these powerful forces in the body was a "fundamentally religious concern." Observers of current chiropractic practice have noted its appeal to those with a spiritual worldview. Homeopathy has similar roots. Its founder, Samuel Hahnemann, believed homeopathy "had unveiled the secret whereby humanity might bring physical events under the action of a 'higher law.'" Today homeopathy offers a vitalistic worldview which encourages a belief that homeopathic remedies act "spiritually" on the material world of the body.

Herbal remedies, fasting, and the varied forms of meditation and hypnosis are all examples of widely used alternative techniques that have explicit religious or spiritual origins. While some practitioners may minimize these spiritual roots, the broader field of alternative medicine actively asserts them. Increasingly there is a recognition that this spiritual dimension is one of alternative medicine's strengths. Unambiguously religious actions, such as prayer for oneself and for others, is increasingly accepted as an alternative healing technique.

Conventional medicine has frequently found it difficult to integrate the role of consciousness, autonomy, and self-control in determining health and illness. The addition of a spiritual dimension implies the inclusion of ideas that are even more remote from the medical mainstream. This includes ideas about the meaning or purpose of life, god, intuition, prayer, collective symbols, myths, and shared responsibility for things like empathy and sacrifice. The equation of health with virtue, and disease with sin, must be reckoned with again.

At the most fundamental level, the incorporation of spirituality into an understanding of health and illness requires confronting basic assumptions about the nature of reality. Is the "real world" limited to the natural world, or is there a supernatural world to contend with as well? If the latter exists, what is the role of rationality in understanding or controlling the world? If there is a supernatural world, it is possible that health, disease, suffering, and the universe itself have meanings beyond the personal—i.e., they may be messages? While contemplating these questions brings comfort to some people, it is acutely distressing to others.

Most hospitals, health insurance companies, medical schools, public health agencies, and other medical institutions are built upon the assumption that the supernatural world is irrelevant to health, illness, and healing. Though many hospitals and medical schools began as religious institutions, with minor exceptions they have left these roots far behind. What are the implications for them of an alternative medicine that is rooted in the supernatural? The implications of a spiritually grounded medicine are equally profound for social norms about health and illness. Do religious and spiritual attitudes and behaviors become key elements in preventing and dealing with illness?

Are some religions better at dealing with illness than others? How can we tell? Does this mean that some religions are "right" (or relatively more "right") while others are "wrong"? If there is an afterlife, what does that imply about the norms and ideals of trying to live a long and healthy life?

As the government pays, directly or indirectly, for most medical care and training in our society, the integration of spiritual matters inevitably leads to conflict-laden questions about the relationship between church and state. What should the government pay for? What should the government prohibit? What about those who are nonbelievers? In sum, the inclusion of a spiritual dimension as essential to understanding the origin of illness and the nature of healing poses a major threat to the nation's dominant medical and political institutions, along with the entire Western scientific understanding of reality.

Spirituality in America

Despite the general assumption of casual observers that the United States has become a secular society, religious and spiritual beliefs remain strong and widespread. These commonly held beliefs are not limited to "liberal" theological notions that view god as a vague and distant force that set the universe in motion and then retired from direct involvement in mundane human affairs. A 1996 national survey of 1,975 representative American adults (excluding Jews, Mormons, and other small groups) carried out by the Pew Research Center for the People and the Press found that 72 percent of all adults were absolutely certain that god exists. Seventy-one percent believe in heaven, 57 percent believe in hell, and 35 percent believe that the Bible is the literal word of god. Almost six of every ten Americans consider religion "very important in their lives," with a similar proportion offering grace at family meals, while about forty percent attend church at least once each week and about thirty percent pray "several times daily." Only about one percent of the adult population admits to being completely atheistic. The Pew Research Center report also noted that religion is a strong and growing force in the way Americans think about politics: "Its increasing influence on political opinion and behavior rival factors such as race, region, age, social class and gender." The annual Gallup Poll, which employs a less restrictive question (belief without being absolutely certain of god's existence), has consistently found well over 90 percent of American adults are believers. These figures have not changed appreciably over the past fifty years. Other polls have typically found that about half the population believe in angels, with somewhat fewer believing in ESP and the existence of devils. Even individuals who profess no specific religious preference frequently engage in prayer and believe in spiritual forces. Likewise, many scientists profess a belief in a god who actively communicates with humans. A 1996 poll of biologists, physicists, and mathematicians found about 40 percent agreed there is a god who can be prayed to "in expectation of receiving an answer." The views of the scientists polled on this matter in 1996 were almost identical to those of scientists who had been polled in 1916, using identical questions. Today, as almost a century ago, only about 15 percent of scientists are willing to call themselves atheists or agnostics.

The religious views of Americans have always informed their ideas about how the body and mind interact, as well as how the supernatural can influence health and illness. While certain groups, such as evangelical Christians, have traditionally voiced spiritual views of health, in the 1990s many more groups are expressing them as well. A 1996 TIME/CNN poll of one thousand four adults representing the U.S. population found a majority believe that personal prayer can have healing power (82 percent), praying for someone else can help cure their illness (73 percent), god sometimes intervenes to cure a serious illness (77 percent), and if patients request it, doctors should join them in prayer (64 percent). A 1982 Gallup Poll estimated that more than eight million Americans have had a "near death" experience, which typically occurs while on the verge of death due to an accident, surgical mishap, or severe illness. The dying individual simultaneously feels peaceful and serene; has an out of body experience (where one leaves one's body and sees it from above); and senses a warm, brilliant, enveloping light ahead through a dark tunnel. Most of those who have this experience report that it leaves them no longer fearing death and enables them to live life to its fullest. The similarity of the experience among the wide range of people who report it has been striking to observers.

Despite the consistency in most broad measures of religious belief, the specific religious views of the American population have recently shifted in some important ways. Since the early 1970s, annual surveys—such as those conducted by the National Opinion Research Center—show that regardless of specific religious preference (and even among those with no preference), Americans have increasingly rejected a view of religion as a source of specific moral absolutes. Simultaneously, they have been coming to value religion as a reflective and spiritual resource. This new outlook on religion is reflected in the specific experiences people report. For example, the respected General Social Survey of the American population carried out by the University of Michigan found that between 1973 and 1988 "mystical experiences" such as deja vu, ESP, and clairvoyance increased due to a higher prevalence among younger people (under sixty years of age). About two thirds of the adult population claim to have personally experienced either "deja vu" (thought you were somewhere you had been before when you knew that was impossible), or ESP (felt you were in touch with someone who was very far away from you). About forty percent of American adults report that they have felt they were in contact with the dead at least once, and a third report they have been "very close to a powerful, spiritual force that seemed to lift you out of yourself."

These surveys combine to depict American culture as one that is already suffused with religious and spiritual beliefs, practices, and experiences. Thus, the emphasis on spirituality within alternative medicine is not at all foreign to a significant proportion of the American population. In fact, it appears that the opposite is true—that now, as in almost every other time in American history, religious beliefs are pivotal to the life experiences of a wide cross-section of American society. If there is any movement away from religion in American society, it appears to be a transition to a less parochial or sectarian approach to decision-making. That is to say, people increasingly rely on religion as a means for self-exploration and reflection and somewhat less frequently as a body of moral doctrine or law. Both the longstanding suffusion of religious and spiritual beliefs throughout American society and this newer emphasis on religion as a spiritual resource make many individuals receptive toward alternative medicine's spiritual connection to health and illness.

Certain alternative approaches encourage individuals to seek a connection with the Divine as a part of maintaining their health or seeking cure from illness. People who believe in a higher power and rely on this relationship to guide them through difficult emotional times are likely to be very comfortable with such a treatment. According to the General Social Survey, 70 percent of Americans reported that when they think of god, the image of a healer is "extremely likely" to come to mind. Another 21 percent of Americans reported the image of god as a healer as "somewhat likely" to come to mind, indicating that 91 percent of the population identifies with the idea of god as a healer. This degree of concordance is remarkable for any area of public opinion. For a large proportion of the American public, then, the emphasis on spirituality in alternative medicine may more fully address their vision of reality than many mainstream approaches.

Science and Spirit

The power of the spirit and religious practice to influence health and illness has not been completely neglected by physicians and mainstream researchers. Beyond many anecdotal accounts, a large and ever growing epidemiologic literature has emerged that consistently supports the salutary effect of religion and religiosity on health. A 1987 review found over 250 published empirical studies that dealt with the topic. The vast majority noted a positive relationship between religious belief or behavior and some specific health outcome. Since that time the literature has grown, with many of the more recent studies employing more sophisticated methods.

An Israeli study that attempted to "determine the association between Jewish religious observance and mortality among study populations with maximal similarity in social structure, social support mechanisms and lifestyle" provides a typical example. The researchers used a historical prospective design and compared rates of mortality over a sixteen-year period in eleven religious and eleven secular kibbutzim. They found that "there was a distinctly lower mortality rate in religious kibbutzim that was evident in both sexes, evident at all ages, and consistent throughout the 16-year period of observation." This lower mortality persisted across the major categories of underlying cause of death. Moreover, "the magnitude of the protective effect associated with membership in a religious kibbutz is exemplified by ablution of the usual female mortality advantage: secular women did not live longer than religious men." Their findings were particularly provocative given the careful attention the authors gave to controlling potential confounding factors. The criteria for "matching" the kibbutzim included "same geographic locale, use of the same regional hospital, similar numbers of members 40 years of age and older, and dates of establishment as close as possible." Furthermore, the researchers controlled for sociodemographic characteristics, including ethnic origin and social class; the "provision, quality and accessibility of primary care services"; and perceived and instrumental social support in their analysis. The authors wrote: "We compared two societies living in almost identical cohesive communal settlements with the same kibbutz ideology of equality and sharing in production and in fulfilling needs." Therefore, the primary difference between the two communities was their religiosity: "Those residing in secular kibbutzim are almost all agnostic or nonreligious, whereas almost all of those residing in religious kibbutzim are religiously orthodox and observant."

As a part of the Kuopio Ischemic Health Disease Risk Factor Study in Finland, researchers examined the relationship between membership in selected religious groups and all-cause mortality in over sixteen hundred men. They controlled for variety of both physiological factors (serum cholesterol, plasma fibrinogen, serum triglycerides, height, weight) and psychosocial variables (income, childhood socioeconomic status, years of education) in the analysis. The researchers found that Eastern Orthodox men had more than five times the mortality than Lutheran men. They concluded that mortality risk varies substantially by religious affiliation and that this variation cannot be attributed to differences in measures for a wide variety of health, behavioral, socioeconomic, biological, and other characteristics. In another study of over five thousand adults, frequent attendees at religious services had considerably lower death rates (24 percent lower for men, 35 percent lower for women) over a twenty-eight-year period than non-attendees with similar health practices and social ties. Other recent research has found that patients who depend on their religious faith are three times as likely to survive open heart surgery, and numerous religious practices are associated with enhanced immune function and a faster recovery from periods of depression and anxiety.

Given the number of studies that have dealt with the topic, and the consistency of the findings, it does seem reasonable to conclude that there is a positive relationship between religious beliefs and behaviors and good health. The questions that remain to be answered are whether the relationship is "real" or valid (not caused by chance or some confounding factor) and whether it is "causal," meaning religiosity actually causes certain health outcomes.

The clear tendency in the academic and research communities has been to accept the validity of the association between religion and health, but also to explain it away as caused by something that doesn't require any belief in the supernatural. Thus, it may be the fact that religious people are less likely to smoke, use drugs, or engage in risky sexual behavior that accounts for their advantage. This perspective is exemplified by a set of studies that found an association between degree of adherence to Mormon Church doctrine and lower lung cancer rates. Others have suggested that there may be some unknown genetic advantage at work, or that religious identity and ritual may be associated with social support which reduces the impact of stress or triggers a physiological immune response. To the extent that any or all of these are accurate, the implication has been that religion is not "really" responsible for the salutary outcome.

Another set of pathways by which religion or religiosity might operate is more specific to religion, but still requires no belief in the supernatural. In this view, religious beliefs produce health by inducing a state of peacefulness, optimism, and calmness, or a nonaggressive stance toward the world. Thus, religion is viewed as a means by which individuals can justify or implement a healthy mental state. Similarly, religious rituals, especially prayer, may bring on various beneficial psychological or physiological states that prevent the onset of illness or reduce its impact in some way. For example, the authors of the kibbutzim study note in their conclusion that "a major possibility is that such a social environment induces less stress, enhances host resistance, and promotes overall well-being and a positive health status." They suggest six possible components of stress reduction specific to membership in an orthodox Jewish kibbutz, none of which are dependent upon the existence of a supernatural reality. Finally, religion, and religious faith, may simply operate as a placebo; it is the believing, not the belief, that is helpful.

Jeff Levin has explored the impact of religion and spirituality on health, along with the myriad ways they might interact. Although a religious believer himself, Levin concludes that the data does not allow any firm conclusion regarding the relationship of religion or spirituality and the *cure* of any illness. He argues that no research on this topic has employed an adequate research design. What does exist is strong evidence that religion and spirituality are useful in the *prevention* of illness or disease in the first place. In epidemiologic terms, religious identity, beliefs, and behaviors contribute to what is called "host resistance" for a wide range of conditions. Although Levin's conclusion that there is no proof religious activity can cure illness may be disappointing to some people, his ideas fit quite nicely with much of the basic alternative belief system: the importance of prevention, the interaction of body and mind, and the understanding of health as the ability to transcend one's limits by conscious effort. After Levin's extensive and well-reasoned review of this large body of research, it is difficult for scholars and clinicians to deny the actual value of religion as a factor in preventing illness and limiting its impact.

Conventional researchers and clinicians are beginning to recognize the religious influence on health and illness. Mainstream researchers have begun to show interest in describing the physiologic correlates of spiritual states on specific organs, such as the eye. Professional associations are including related topics in their journals and meetings. For example, the American Society of Clinical Oncology had a formal symposium on spiritual factors in cancer survival at its 1996 annual meeting that recognized spirituality as the predominant long-term coping mechanism most people actually use for dealing with cancer. Thus, there is evidence that conventional medicine is beginning to include religion and spirituality in the study of health and illness. But, for the most part, mainstream providers try to understand these factors in terms of the dominant naturalistic biomedical paradigm.

Some researchers are attempting to understand the relationship of religion or spirit and health outside of the conventional biomedical paradigm. The best known and most well articulated of these efforts has been the work of a physician, Larry Dossey, who has used developments in modern physics as a means of integrating spirituality and health. Dossey's work details scores of studies whose findings of healing would appear irreconcilable with a scientific understanding of reality. They include examples of healing without using any known means of physical intervention, but rather through the intentional mental or "psychic" influence of a person (or persons) on a living organism. For example, Dossey cites the work of Daniel Benor who examined 131 controlled trials and experiments in which people used their thoughts to manipulate the physical characteristics of enzymes, cells, plants, animals, and other humans. Seventy-seven of these studies had statistically significant positive results.

Dossey's work offers the "new physics," with its concept of "nonlocal" events, as a possible means of explaining these results. The great attraction of such explanations is that they enable prayer as well as shamanistic and psychic healing to be understood within a naturalistic view of the universe. It is mainstream medicine that now becomes "unscientific" if it refuses to incorporate these post-Newtonian views. In essence, Dossey and others are saying that if one believes in empirical science, one must recognize the accumulation of good data that is not explainable by traditional mainstream science. The choices for medicine are either to accept a supernatural explanation for these findings, or look to recent developments in the basic sciences that now offer a possible set of explanations. Adopting the latter stance will enable clinicians to create a "nonlocal medicine," which will allow them to do what is best for their patients, such as praying for them or with them, while avoiding or "bridging" the god issue.

Dossey describes what he sees as three eras of medicine. Era I medicine is based solely upon traditional mechanistic ideas about space and time. Mind is not a factor in Era I medicine, and therapy consists of drugs or procedures that have a direct impact on the body. Era II is "mind-body medicine" where the mind operates within an individual. Era II therapies include imagery, PNI, etc. Era III "nonlocal or transpersonal" medicine uses the mind to bring about healing both within and between people. "Mind is unbounded and infinite in space and time—thus omnipresent, eternal, and ultimately unitary or one." In Era III, treatments such as therapeutic touch, shamanism, intercessory prayer, and telepathy now become part of medicine. Dossey even foresees a future where prayer will become such an accepted part of medical interventions that its absence in a treatment plan would be grounds for a malpractice suit.

At this time, the mechanism through which religious belief affects health status is unresolved. It has, nonetheless, been brought to the epidemiological research agenda and is now recognized as relevant to the future of our thinking about health and illness. If religion operates through naturalistic mechanisms, then it is in the public interest to design interventions that enhance access to those mechanisms for both religious and nonreligious individuals. If the power of religious belief and affiliation lies beyond naturalist explanations, society may have to grapple with the most fundamental issues about the nature of health and illness. Despite the ambiguity and controversy that characterize the state of the literature at this time, there already are enough studies indicating a robust relationship between religion and health to both empower advocates of the alternative perspective and threaten mainstream practitioners.

Of course, there are any number of physicians, clergy, and clients who see no need to explain, reconcile, or justify the findings of studies indicating that prayer or spirituality influences health. For these individuals, god—the supernatural explanation—is perfectly acceptable. But this is a view that neither the majority of conventional nor alternative practitioners find most comfortable.

Conventional Medicine's Response

Mainstream medicine's response to alternative medicine has traditionally been ambivalent, at best. In recent years, the tone of scorn and hostility that characterized the "official" views of organized medicine have become considerably muted. Today, Western medicine is considerably more open to alternative approaches and appreciates the limits of many conventional techniques. Still, it is clear that one of the most problematic qualities of an alternative perspective is the inclusion of spirituality as an essential aspect of healing.

One dimension of the conventional medical community's response to the inclusion of spirituality when dealing with illness is exemplified by a "sounding board" essay in the *New England Journal of Medicine*. This article asserted that conventional medicine is a "form of consultant engineering" and criticized the notion that physicians should also act as "consolers." While the authors saw the latter as logically tenable, if misguided, they considered doctors taking on a spiritual personality to be a logically impossible combination of roles. Calling the "banal rhetoric about the physician as consoler" a "deliberate attempt to substitute a magical for an engineering conception of the physician and an attack on scientific understanding and reason," they described spiritually informed alternative approaches as "a pabulum of common sense and nonsense offered by cranks and quacks and failed pedants who share an attachment to magic and an animosity toward reason." The essay is lengthy and scathing. But the *NEJM*'s decision to publish it as an "opinion piece" makes it clear that there is some ambivalence toward its conclusions.

A 1991 flap involving *JAMA* revealed a similar set of mixed feelings toward spirituality from the medical community. An article by Deepak Chopra and two other self-described Ayurvedic physicians set out what they believed to be the contributions of Ayurvedic medicine. The article went through *JAMA*'s full peer review process. But when concerns were raised about the links of the authors, especially Chopra, to Maharishi Mahesh Yogi and Transcendental Meditation (TM), *JAMA* backtracked. The editor wrote a "correction/clarification" and published a seven-page response, which criticized the authors of the article for withholding full financial disclosure information and detailed allegations against the Maharishi, his practices, organizations, and ideology. The response called TM a "cult" which promotes the belief that it can end all war, make people invisible, and enable them to walk through walls and fly through the air. Much of *JAMA*'s hostile response was supposedly generated by the fear that Chopra and the other authors might be in a position to benefit financially from any increase in TM's popularity. Yet the authors of many clinical reports in medical journals about drugs and other interventions stand to benefit financially from positive findings. It is clear that the association of positive findings with a particular set of spiritual views was the source of discomfort and controversy within the medical establishment.

JAMA's response to the Chopra article illustrates mainstream medicine's tendency to label spiritual or religious views as "anti-science." The idealized scientific worldview is presented as being objective and based upon universalistic quantifiable criteria, rationality, and skepticism. The anti-science worldview, on the other hand, is epitomized as subjective, qualitative, nonfalsifiable, equally accessible to everyone, and spiritual in the values it promotes. From this perspective, an attack upon mainstream medicine's neglect of spirituality can be seen as the embodiment of some larger assault on science, rationality, and the structure of modern society. The implicit assumption is that spiritual and religious practices and techniques may be relatively harmless in themselves. But when they are allowed to enter into existing medical institutions and organizations, they have the potential to create great havoc.

But the attitudes that underlie organized medicine's response toward increasing spirituality in medical practice is only partially reflected by articles like the *JAMA* response to Chopra or the *NEJM* "sounding board." There is a growing acceptance of the idea that health care professionals themselves, within mainstream medicine, have spiritual needs that should be addressed. The very nature of medical work leads to stress, tension, and burnout. These problems are most likely to effect those who deal with clients who are either very ill or require long-term assistance to lead healthier lifestyles. This is difficult work, which under the current move toward managed care has become even more time limited and stressful. In this context, research has begun to describe the salutary impact of spiritual involvement on health care providers themselves. For example, Carol Montgomery found that spiritual transcendence was the main reason nurses were able to avoid burnout. Spirituality gave the nurses more energy, helped them make better connections with their patients, and left them feeling less depressed by setbacks to their patients. Experiencing god as a source of energy was the key to being able to provide a sense of caring. These findings support the earlier work of June Lowenberg that the combination of caring, compassion, and spirituality enabled many types of practitioners (M.D.s, R.N.s, and others) to be able to encourage clients with AIDS to assume more personal responsibility for their actions, while not "blaming" them for their disease or condition.

There is a growing recognition that intimate experiences, training, and clinical expertise affect how doctors understand illness and behave toward patients. My own earlier studies comparing members of the American Holistic Medical Association and conventional family physicians showed that the alternative doctors are much more likely to be aware of how their own spiritual experiences and personal bouts with illness have shaped their professional lives. It was their worldviews, as opposed to the clinical attitudes and practices, that distinguished the groups from one another. As American society becomes more accepting of a spiritual connection to health, conventional physicians may be more likely to follow suit.

Turning Religion into Medicine

The religious and spiritual roots of alternative medicine are deep and strong. The mass of the American populace is strongly favorable toward religion and spirituality. A large body of research indicates that religious commitments and behavior are beneficial for one's health. But the institutions that comprise the medical mainstream, and most physicians themselves, are skeptical of integrating spirituality, no less religion, into medicine. This is the dilemma facing alternative medicine as it becomes a part of the contemporary medical landscape.

In large part, alternative medicine has dealt with this skepticism by deemphasizing or renaming its religious roots and commitments. Sometimes these linkages are simply downplayed as historical remnants (as in the case of chiropractic) or even hidden. The assumption is that the technique or approach to healing can stand on its own; its religious origins are largely irrelevant. Thus, a widely cited compendium of alternative therapies extols fasting as "a low cost, effective therapy for a wide range of conditions, including hypertension, headaches, allergies, and arthritis" but says nothing about fasting's religious origins. But this example of masked religious origins is atypical. For the most part, contemporary alternative medicine deals with its sectarian religious roots by reclassifying them as "spiritual."

Such efforts at relabeling are not new. Robert Fuller has described in great detail how a very similar pattern of "spiritualizing" took place among healers in the late nineteenth century, when "America was awash in 'irregular,' sectarian healing systems, among them homeopathy, Thomsonianism, hydropathy, and sundry dietary regimens. . . . All of these resonated with the . . . perfectionist tendencies of early nineteenth century American Protestantism." Fuller offers a detailed account of how the work of Mesmer provided the concept of "animal magnetism," which explained how the integration of the body's matter, mind, and spirit could take place. The animal magnetism concept represented a relabeling of religious ideas into a more accessible notion. While animal magnetism was compatible with Christianity, it also appealed to "those whose religious sensibilities could not be constrained by scriptural piety and who yearned for a progressive, co-scientific religious outlook." Ideas like animal magnetism viewed god not as a problematic "thing" or entity, but as a force in nature, which is controlled by our minds. The mind has the power to control how things in nature (food, contact with fresh air) can make contact with our inner physical bodies. Thus, something like diet or exercise takes on a spiritual quality in that it is a vehicle for god's presence. This connection, which Fuller calls "spiritualizing," is a common part of alternative medicine.

Contemporary alternative medicine is filled with examples of a sectarian "god" being turned into a nonsectarian "spirit." The relationship is similar to that promoted in Alcoholics Anonymous (AA). AA demands the alcoholic turn him or herself over to a "higher power." This phrase explicitly requires a "god," but AA is equally explicit that everyone is free to define "god" however they choose. In practice, a nonsectarian spiritualism prevails with the group accepting however each individual member understands god. AA's approach has been widely adopted by hundreds of other self-help groups, some explicitly and others implicitly. The widespread prevalence of such groups, and their (perceived) success in dealing with all sorts of seemingly intractable problems, has popularized the replacement of religious with spiritual beliefs. The adoption of a diffuse, individualized spiritualism also has the advantage of making a group or technique accessible to a broad range of participants, many of whom might not be as comfortable with a more focused and specific set of beliefs. As documented by Robert Bellah and his associates in their book *Habits of the Heart*, most strata of American society are filled with people who describe themselves as "not religious" but spiritual.

In a society where belief in god is so widespread, it should not be surprising that many people intensely desire integrating religion and spirituality into health care. Serious illness and thoughts of mortality intensify people's desire to seek meaning in their lives. Mainstream medicine has become increasingly deficient in its ability to offer meaning to those who are ill, and the rise of managed care has exacerbated this gap. With its emphasis on energy forces uniting the individual's body and mind, alternative medicine is very much like "Eastern mystical traditions, which deny any sharp distinction between spirit and matter and portray God as a spiritual energy continuously exerting causal influences within the physical universe."

For many consumers and providers, the ability of alternative medicine to convert sectarian religion into a diffuse nonsectarian spirituality is a great attraction. For most people confronting and living with serious illness, their condition marks a major transformation in life. Spirituality and religion, and the practices they encompass, can be great resources for dealing with these crises. A good deal of the success of people like Deepak Chopra, Shakti Gawain, and Jon Kabat-Zinn lies in their ability to make the teachings of ancient religious traditions (Ayurveda, Tibetan meditative practice, and Zen Buddhism, respectively) more accessible and acceptable to an educated American audience. They do this by selectively emphasizing basic spiritual precepts. Alternative medicine offers individuals a nonsectarian spiritual framework that both validates the inclusion of religion and spirituality in health and healing and makes specific practices more available to mainstream American society.

One of the most well known advocates of a "dereligicized" understanding of spirit as a means of improving health and healing is Herbert Benson. Over twenty years ago, Benson, a physician, was writing about the placebo effect as a "neglected asset" of medicine. Since then his work has documented the power of the placebo effect over the widest variety of conditions. His best selling book, *The Relaxation Response,* promotes a meditative technique derived from Transcendental Meditation (itself a highly Westernized and secularized approach to meditation) with almost no overt "religious" content. The technique is presented as having two major "selling points": (1) its documented impact on a range of physiologic functions such as respiration and blood pressure and (2) its simplicity and nonsectarian character, which make it accessible to anyone. Benson himself describes his technique as a demystified form of meditation. In his most recent book, *Timeless Healing: The Power and Biology of Belief,* Benson explicitly brings the spiritual dimension back: "Faith quiets the mind like no other form of belief. . . . Because faith seems to transcend experience and base reality, it is supremely good at quieting distress and generating hope and expectancy. With hope and expectancy comes remembered wellness—the neurosignature messages of healing that mobilize the body's resources and reactions." His emphasis on the spiritual dimension of healing includes any and all religious traditions (as well as none at all): "Regardless of how traditional one's practice of religious beliefs, whenever faith is present, remembered wellness is triggered and health can be improved." Benson explicitly endorses religious ritual as health-enhancing: "Remembered wellness makes the religious ritual a very powerful mechanism. There is something very influential about invoking a ritual that may have first been practiced in childhood, about regenerating the neural pathways that were formed in your youthful experience of faith." Benson offers a naturalistic explanation for his findings: "Perhaps this tendency of human beings to worship and believe was rooted in our physiology, written into our genes, encoded in our very make-up. . . . I suspect that belief in God is a primal motive or a survival instinct." However, his conclusions clearly have spiritual implications: "My scientific studies have . . . conclusively shown that our bodies are wired to believe, that our bodies are nourished and healed by prayer and other exercises of belief." He urges readers, "Let faith, the ultimate belief, heal you."

The transformation of religious meditation into secularized meditation and eventually a "relaxation response" is similar to the conversion of the "laying on of hands" into "Therapeutic Touch." Like the relaxation response, Therapeutic Touch is a trademarked term. It refers to the use of sweeping graceful movements of the hands a few inches away from the body of the patient. Its advocates claim it can replenish the flow of energy in the patient, remove obstructions and congestion, and restore balance to the energy flow within the body. It is promoted as a method of "healing," not merely "curing," that grants relief beyond whatever power it may have as a placebo.

A similar secularized version of ancient religious healing techniques can be seen in the "8 Week Self Balancing Plan" being popularized by Andrew Weil in book form as well as through his appearances on television and his website on the

Internet. Each week participants are given a number of things to do. For the first week these include "throw out all animal fat" and "eat more fruit," along with the injunction to "sit quietly every day for five minutes and listen attentively to your breathing." Just as the dietary and exercise components of the plan become increasingly rigorous over the eight weeks, the "spiritual" instructions move participants toward meditation ("sit quietly and breathe slowly," "do eight slow breathing repetitions twice a day"), and removing oneself from the concerns of material life ("spend two days a week without reading, watching, or listening to the news," "visit an art museum," "spend time listening to music"). The explicit notion is that one can be spiritual without being religious: "Many people consider spirit to be in the province of religion, but I insist on making a clear distinction between spirituality and religion. Spirituality has to do with the nonphysical, immaterial aspects of our beings—with energies, essences, and the parts of us that existed before and will exist after the disintegration of the body. . . . *It is possible to lead a spiritual life and explore the influence of spirituality on health whether you are religious or not.*"

When Weil speaks of his program he emphasizes the role of spirituality: "Human beings are bodies, minds, spirits. Health necessarily involves all of these components and any program intended to improve health must address all of them." He exhorts his readers to include spiritual concerns in their healing process: "To optimize the function of the healing system you must do everything in your power to improve physical health, mental/emotional health, and spiritual health." The message on his homepage is the same: "In my world view optimum health isn't just fitness. It's well being of body, mind, and spirit." At the same time, Weil clearly believes that there is a connection between religion and healing. A decade earlier he wrote that "medicine, religion, and science are rooted in common ideas, and each sheds light on the other. But the supremacy of scientific technology makes it fashionable to believe that medicine has nothing to do with such old fashioned practices as religion and magic. Consequently, many modern doctors cannot grasp the true meaning of health. . . ."

Larry Dossey, the executive editor of *Alternative Therapies* as well as the author of a number of widely read books on the spiritual aspects of alternative medicine, has commented most explicitly on the tension and ambiguity involved in bringing religious action into the practice of medicine. Throughout his writing Dossey draws on the empirical literature (beyond case reports) that documents attempts to use "prayer" to bring about healing. The importance and influence of his work comes from his model of prayer as a "nonlocal phenomena" that arises from human action and does not require any belief in god. For Dossey, prayer is not some sort of energy that is "sent" to someone or somewhere. He views prayer as "information" that is infinite in time and space. Thus, it has nowhere to go, and an external god is irrelevant. The divine is already within us, in what he terms a "modern" model of prayer. Dossey claims that this "nonlocal" phenomenon has been scientifically proven to exist. The proof he offers emerges from physics which has documented that if "distant objects have once been in contact, a change thereafter in one causes an immediate change in the other—no matter how far apart they are, even if they are separated to the opposite ends of the universe. [This] is not just a theoretical idea in physics; it rests on actual experiments."

Once scientific law can explain prayer, it becomes easy to explain all sorts of things: anecdotes, experimental findings about the work of healers and physicians, and the conclusions of epidemiologists about the importance of religion for health. Dossey doesn't view prayer as a panacea; it is a weak force in the universe, hard to mobilize and direct. Indeed, Dossey believes that nondirected prayer is twice as effective as prayer directed toward a specific outcome. Of course, the fact that such prayers have, by definition, no desired outcome makes it difficult to evaluate their use. Still, Dossey sees the use of prayer becoming an increasingly important part of the medical armamentarium. Dossey's explicit goal is to "recover the soul" and "the power of prayer" for a nonsectarian contemporary medicine.

Turning Medicine into Religion

In most societies throughout history, religion and the healing arts have been intimately connected. In this regard, the separation of medicine and religion in the United States over the past several decades has been an aberration. Perhaps the best way to understand the rising popularity of using spirituality to understand illness is to simply view it as a reassertion of this traditional connection. Dossey writes, "Contagious magic seems woven into the fabric of the universe! . . . Could humans be joined in much the same eerie way that subatomic particles are connected, and could this connectedness make possible negative prayer and distant hexing? . . . *Whether this makes God the ultimate practitioner of contagious magic is an interesting question.*" There is little difference between Dossey's ideas and those set out by D. D. Palmer or Ellen White in their early works on chiropractic and Seventh Day Adventism.

A similar blending of spirituality with medicine is easy to find in the work of most well known exponents of alternative medicine. For example, Kenneth Pelletier's influential book, *Holistic Medicine,* validated the core assumptions of alternative medicine by placing them within the context of the then emerging field of psychosomatic medicine. But his "new paradigm" is infused with pure religion and spirituality and offers "knowing thyself" as the "ultimate exercise," along with "a quest for perfectibility" as the "highest manifestation of a great design." Dean Ornish concluded a description of his program to reverse coronary disease by saying: "So these are very old ideas. The ancient swamis and rabbis and priests and monks and nuns who developed these techniques didn't develop them to unclog their arteries or lower their cholesterol or blood pressure. They developed them because they helped to quiet their mind and body, and give them direct experience that on one level we're all separate—you are you and I'm me—and on another level we're part of something larger that connects us all."

David Reilly is a Scottish physician, best known in the alternative medical community for publishing data from a randomized control study in the *Lancet* that supported the use of homeopathy to treat allergies. But Reilly himself believes that his patients who consult him as a shaman, seeking presence and wisdom, get better results than those who use him as a homeopath. His "most satisfying moment" as a practitioner comes when his patients reject a homeopathic remedy because they've been "touched." He writes, "I do homeopathy. But that doesn't matter very much. The religion, the medicine, the bits and the bobs. In the end, we're just human beings."

The voices of Chopra, Siegel, Pelletier, Cousins, and dozens of others offer us contemporary versions of the same themes that Graham, Mesmer, Palmer, and many others offered in the nineteenth century. Just as these early advocates grounded their religious views in the latest science of the day, Dossey and others seek to recast religion and spirituality in the up-to-date vocabulary of post-Einsteinian physics. Since much of the American population has always held religious beliefs independent of any deep identity with a particular set of dogma or church membership, even the nonsectarian nature of the spirituality expounded within alternative medicine is not new.

The overt and at times overarching religion and spirituality in alternative medicine meets with frequent hostility from mainstream medicine. Many practitioners view it as a reflection of the general population's ignorance of science, as well as a form of resistance to the control and influence exerted by an educated, scientifically literate elite. The potential impact of a scientifically illiterate populace on public policy regarding the funding of medical research or health services is often upsetting to conventional physicians and their institutions. In a scathing critique of the growing anti-science sentiment, Gerald Holton quotes Dostoevsky in *The Brothers Karamozov*: "No science will give the masses bread so long as they remain free. In the end they will lay their freedom at our feet and say to us: 'Make us slaves, but feed us.' . . . There are three powers, three powers alone, able to conquer and hold captive forever the conscience of these impotent rebels for their happiness—those forces are miracle, mystery, and authority." Most disturbing to conventional physicians and scientists is the notion, frequently expressed by many in the alternative medical community, that as scientific concepts and categories are all creations of the human mind, there is no true distinction between fact and fiction. Commenting on his decision to write *The Return of Merlin*, Chopra noted that nonfiction leaves people saying "where is the evidence? And it's so boring to try to address that! [But] if you write fiction . . . with intensity and passion, you reveal yourself—and you write the truth. . . ." When someone like Deepak Chopra, trained in the Western scientific tradition, turns to writing novels as a means of more accurately portraying the reality of what causes illness and its cure, critics can easily interpret this as an all-out attack on a rational understanding of nature. The use of quantification and concepts (e.g., atoms or microbes) that are not part of commonsense experience, as well as the fundamental secularism of Western society, are threatened. In this context, advocacy of alternative medicine becomes nothing less than a form of Ludditism that attacks the rationality, objectivity, cosmopolitanism, and individualism of modern society itself.

In place of a world where increased rationality is supposed to lead to a better life, the anti-science perspective offers a spiritual and ecstatic return to nature—what critics Paul Gross and Norman Levitt called "the Gates of Eden." The search for "Eden" tells us to reject science and technology, instead putting our hope in nature and spirit, and adopt a secure recognition that life is purposive. In this view just as scientific "progress" is seen as inevitably leading to pollution and the despoliation of the physical and social world, medical "progress" inevitably results in iatrogenic illness, and the destruction of our natural ways of healing. According to Gross, Levitt, and many within the medical profession, such views are nothing more than superstitious nonsense that signifies a return to pre-scientific mentality.

Those who represent a conventional religious point of view have also been critical of much of the spirituality in alternative medicine. To many religious people, the very idea of "nonsecular" spirituality is offensive. Alternative medicine typically makes a "crucial presupposition" that "society is now secular and interpretations of spirituality should—indeed must—reflect this." Alternative medicine offers a new "orthodoxy" that separates the spiritual from the religious and makes the former a personal search for meaning. "The concept of God is generally excluded and so becomes marginal and virtually insignificant." In alternative medicine, a comparative religious perspective is dominant, with the assumption that all religions are equally valid. Individuals simply need to choose the one, ones, or bits and pieces of each that suit them best. Over the past few decades the voices of religion have sought to be more fully heard and recognized within the institutions of conventional medical practice. While on a superficial level alternative medicine would appear to be more responsive to these concerns, the institutional religious community remains, at best, ambivalent towards it.

Commentators such as Christopher Lasch and Ivan Illich, who advocate the progressive view that religion is a force to combat the savages of industrial capitalism, have raised a somewhat similar set of criticisms about the role of spirituality in alternative medicine. Such critics consider the overriding problem for modern societies to be the destruction of traditional institutions by advanced industrial capitalism. The family and the church are two important institutions whose power to protect individuals from the onslaughts of industrialization have been largely emasculated. Each of these authors has seen medical institutions as providing a very weak substitute for the protection traditionally offered by the family or religion. Each has sought to imbue religion with a renewed sense of authority in order to help limit capitalism's destruction of crucial human values. From this perspective, the inclusion of spirituality and "nonsectarian" prayer or ritual as a part of medicine is most unwelcome. It exemplifies the ultimate triumph of what Illich calls the "medical nemesis," or the ability of medical terms and values to rob people of their humanity.

Spirituality's Impact on the Future of Alternative Medicine

Given its central and pronounced role, what impact will spirituality have on the future of alternative medicine? Will the immense pool of spiritual and religious feeling among the population facilitate the integration of alternative approaches into the medical mainstream? Or will the emphasis upon spirituality prove to be an unbridgeable gap with mainstream medical institutions in the context of a pluralistic, democratic, industrial society?

Clearly, the spiritual dimension that pervades alternative medicine is one of its great strengths and attractions. There is a widespread recognition that healing is facilitated by an element of "magic," along with the application of knowledge about the body, mind, and techniques of therapy. Any healer, or type of healing, that can give a sense of hope and meaning to symptoms and illness will be more apt to succeed than one that cannot. At the very least, it will be well thought of by those who use it. Much of conventional medicine has failed in this regard. A large component of alternative medicine's success has been its ability to offer a sense of spirituality that, for many people, allows some "magic" to enter the healing process. Without its spiritual dimension, alternative medicine would be a vastly different phenomenon. The vital importance of healing as a source of meaning simply cannot be under-estimated. Dossey put it this way in an exhortation to physicians: "Much of society's disillusionment with modern medicine lies in its failure to acknowledge the importance of meaning in health. . . . The contest between conventional and alternative medicine is not about economics, efficacy, safety, and availability; it is about meaning. . . . No matter how technologically effective modern medicine may be, if it does not honor the place of meaning in illness it may lose the allegiance of those it serves."

Meaning is the central issue in comprehending mind-body interaction. A "healer" is someone who can change consciousness and alter meaning. Consciousness itself, in large measure, is meaning. The absence of meaning, if not the equivalent of illness, promotes and intensifies illness. Throughout history, religion and spirituality have been the major means by which meaning is altered. Conventional medicine and physicians have frequently neglected, forgotten, or rejected this reality. It is this glaring gap, be it one of omission or commission, that offers alternative approaches and practitioners their major point of entry to those who are seriously ill.

The contemporary practice of conventional medicine is more accepting or at least more open to spirituality and "meaning" within medical practice than it has been in the recent past. The photograph in *Life Magazine* of a healer creating an aura over a patient in surgery, working jointly with a surgeon, described in the fourth paragraph of this book, is a vivid and dramatic example of this new openness. But, more mundane evidence exists as well. A recent survey of three hundred family practice physicians found that 99 percent believed a patient's religious beliefs could have a positive effect upon the healing process, and 80 percent believed that prayer and meditation have palliative power. The vast majority of these physicians actively sought to integrate these spiritual elements into their practices. Increasingly such sentiments are finding a response in continuing education programs for physicians. Each year since 1995, the Harvard Medical School's Department of Continuing Education has held a course entitled "Spirituality and Healing in Medicine" that has drawn over a thousand attendees annually. The sessions have included talks on Hindu, Buddhist, Jewish, Catholic, Islamic, Pentecostal, Christian Science, and Seventh Day Adventist healing practices. Many talks are offered by practicing clergy, not academics or scholars. For example, a talk on Christian Science was given by Virginia Harris, chairman of the Christian Science Board of Directors. The course organizer, Dr. Herbert Benson, noted that he now gets five or six calls a week from HMOs that want to incorporate relaxation and other nontraditional healing techniques into their programs. Benson believes that it is unnecessary to differentiate between psychological and spiritual interventions. He finds about 80 percent of his clients are most comfortable with prayer. "So," he writes, "I found I was teaching prayer."

Growing numbers of conventionally trained physicians, especially those in family or primary care medicine, are calling for a "reinvention" of medical practice to encompass the spiritual. The physician is exhorted to view patients' symptoms or complaints within a perspective that includes a spiritual dimension. The idea of healing is expanded to include restoring a sense of internal balance, increasing awareness, and developing a sense of wholeness and meaning, along with any physiological and symptomatic changes. Thus, healing without spirituality is impossible. As Richard Friedman, a professor of psychiatry and participant at the Harvard Conference noted, "Let me make a prediction. Ten years from now . . . doctors will not only ask for a medical history when you come in, but will routinely ask about your belief system as well." In 1995 only a handful of American medical schools offered formal course work on religion and spirituality. By 1998 over thirty did.

In a way that would have seemed impossible if not bizarre a few years ago, conventional medical researchers are beginning to take up the challenge of integrating spirituality into clinical practice. At Duke University, the Department of Medicine is doing randomized, blind, controlled trials of intercessory prayers for 150 patients undergoing cardiac catheterization. Half the patients in the study are being prayed for by up to 100 strangers in eight religious groups around the world: Moravians, Baptists, Carmelite nuns, Buddhist monks in Nepal and France, Jews in Jerusalem, and others. The researchers will be looking at post-operative pain, recovery time, and many other outcomes.

Despite such accounts, the integration of spirituality into conventional medicine is far from well established. Neither is it always considered desirable or feasible, even by those who generally support it. Little is known about whether most conventional practitioners are able to effectively convey spiritual techniques to their clients, or whether the clients will be receptive to their inclusion. It is also difficult to assess whether specific spiritual techniques can be adopted by conventional practitioners without adopting the underlying principles upon which they are based. This is of particular concern with regard to techniques, such as TCM, that emerge directly from Taoism and Confucianism. The central tenets of these faiths focus on how to live a balanced life, how to best relate to other people, and how to adopt a "proper" style of life. Can the doctor as moral teacher be integrated into our image of the doctor as purveyor of scientific knowledge and technical intervention? Do clients really want, or will they accept, moral advice in lieu of or alongside diagnoses, prescriptions, and therapy? Dossey has written what amounts to a guide to prayer for people who are sick. He accepts that prayer styles will vary according to one's temperament or personality. But, on the basis of empirical studies (The Spindrift experiments), he advocates "nondirected" prayer (prayer without a specific goal) as more effective. Yet Dossey realizes that the use of nondirected prayer as a response to ill health is difficult for many people. Users may have a hidden agenda such as, "I'll pray nondirectly, but I wouldn't mind a cure." Dossey himself is comfortable with the notion that prayer "works" when it leads to a new understanding of the meaning of life or some other new experience or struggle. But will most patients and physicians feel the same?

A crucial question is to what extent the assumptions of an alternative medicine that values spirituality, god, surrender, inner peace, and a clear (if not necessarily conventional) moral code can be integrated into the world of mainstream medicine that is built upon scientific rationality, emotional and intellectual distance from the client, and economic self interest.

Today, when so much of medicine and health care is intimately tied up with the government, these issues have become increasingly complex. Currently the government, directly or indirectly, pays for more than half of the nation's health care expenditures. This includes Medicaid, Medicare, medical research, public health agencies and hospitals, the Veterans Administration hospitals and clinics, and various tax subsidies. The government is also instrumental in setting standards of care; prioritizing research; paying for medical education; and dealing with the widest range of health emergencies, from floods and other natural disasters to pollution and epidemics. All of this takes place within the constitutionally mandated separation of church and state. Although the precise meaning of "the separation of church and state" is constantly being reinterpreted through the courts, it is difficult to imagine that integrating many of alternative medicine's core beliefs about the role of spirituality into mainstream medicine would go unchallenged. The list of legal and policy issues is long and daunting: Could government funds pay for doctors to "teach" people to pray? Could medical education include instruction in religious belief and prayer? Would prayer be offered for all conditions, or just those that are chronic, terminal, psychosomatic, or unresponsive to standard biomedicine? How might such care be evaluated? Would failure mean that the patient just hadn't prayed "hard enough," or might it be a sign of unworthiness? The integration of spirituality into a given individual's response to illness, or a single provider's response to illness, may be desirable and beneficial. However, the institutionalization of these ideas within the health care system is likely to create intense conflict.

The centrality of the separation of church and state in American society, and the unintended consequences of injecting spirituality and religion as significant components of the health care system, cannot be underestimated. In this regard, analogies from the field of education may be useful. On the one hand, there is significant although far from universal support for bringing religion and spirituality into publicly funded education. Some people support vouchers that would offer government funds for parochial schools. But most people do not support these programs, and the issue is hotly debated. A somewhat larger portion of the populace supports the inclusion of some religious content, such as the Ten Commandments, in the public school curricula. But, again, a large proportion does not, or disagrees about what should be included or what should be taught about whatever is included. As a practical matter, the only true consensus is over purely symbolic matters such as the inclusion of the phrase "under God" in the Pledge of Allegiance, as long as students have the choice to remain silent when it is said. Would the situation in medicine be much different?

Advocates like Dossey and others appear to be naive about the difficulties that integrating spirituality poses for the American health care system. While health and illness are intimate and private events, medical care and, to a large degree, prevention have become community or public events. Dealing with illness takes place in public and quasi-public institutions, or within private institutions that are largely dependent on government funds. Care is delivered by professionals trained and certified by the government and largely paid for by public funds. When errors are committed, the option exists for people to seek remediation in the courts, through malpractice suits. The inclusion of spirituality, which for most people is tied to religion, poses a major challenge to the entire institutional structure of American medicine.

Conflict over the inclusion of spirituality in medicine has already begun. In January of 1996, the U.S. Supreme Court affirmed a lower court ruling that awarded $1.5 million to a father whose son had died after being treated for diabetes by a Christian Science practitioner engaged by the child's mother and stepfather. The mother, stepfather, and two Christian Science practitioners were held liable for the money. At the least, this precedent sends a chilling message to those who seek to expand the use of prayer in the treatment and cure of illness. If people can be sued for practicing their religion, all sorts of possibilities may be imagined. It has already been suggested that government funding for research on the use of prayer to alleviate illness may violate the Constitution and make the state liable.

The historic identification of American society as a "melting pot" containing a wide diversity of religious, ethnic, and racial groups exacerbates these issues still more. While advocates like Dossey can stress their view that any and all religions or styles of prayer are equally valid, the social reality of American life will not necessarily conform. In Los Angeles County alone there are eighty-six different languages spoken in the public schools. Many of these are representative of different ethnic and religious groups, each of which has its own strongly held ideas about what constitutes the "right way of praying." Will all be equally accepted and integrated into the health care system? Should native healers be made available, at public expense, for each group so that spirituality is equally accessible? What about all those people who wish to assimilate and discard their traditional beliefs? What about atheists and agnostics? Is "equal" treatment possible for them? If prayer is so important for healing, perhaps atheism or the refusal to pray should be regarded as "noncompliance" with treatment or malingering. Even now these questions are not purely hypothetical. Screening instruments have already been developed to help physicians distinguish which of their patients would benefit most from spiritual interventions. Thus, one's spiritual history or potential to be spiritual is now viewed by some researchers and clinicians as a risk factor, to be used in assessing who should receive certain treatments.

Traditionally, most healers have practiced in homogenous communities and shared many of the beliefs of their patients. What happens when this is no longer the case? In America the diversity of views and values between individuals is immense. The very fabric of the society, and one of the hallmarks of its success, is the creation of norms and institutions that transcend this diversity. Much of what is powerful in alternative medicine has emerged from religious traditions that are not widely held in America. Most medical institutions—such as hospitals, medical schools, and insurance companies—are built upon assumptions about the separation of the material and spiritual worlds. Worldviews, particularly those arising from Eastern and other traditional religions that assume a unified world, itself only a reflection of reality, may simply prove to be too remote to be usefully integrated into this structure. On the other hand, Eastern religions often suppose a monistic universe. They teach the ultimately illusory quality of the physical world, the inherent divinity of humans, and the possibility of intrapsychic connections between people. Monistic religions generally have a minimal emphasis on moral absolutism. They tend to avoid "fixed moral codes and rites of confession and atonement." This style differs dramatically from the pentecostal and evan-

gelical movements with their strident affirmation of moral absolutes regarding good and evil and their apocalyptic visions.
In this regard, the nonjudgmental spirituality of alternative
medicine may lend itself more easily to integration into mainstream medical institutions and the minds of those already suffering from illness and disability. As Chopra characterized it,
"They say you have to give up everything to be spiritual, get
away from the world, all that junk. I satisfy a spiritual yearning
without making people think they have to worry about God
and punishment."

5 Is There *Really* an Alternative Medicine?

There is a set of core beliefs that conceptually unifies the wide range of alternative techniques and approaches. But how does alternative medicine manifest itself in the real world? When viewed over time, it is clear that alternative medicine is emerging as an actual reality in terms of practitioners' cooperation in joint ventures and shared identity, as well as in the response of the larger society. The degree of cohesiveness, solidarity, and interaction is greater than ever before and is growing rapidly. This can be seen in the swiftly increasing number of joint activities in which different types of alternative practitioners seek to create a common set of educational experiences and in the growth of professional associations and publications. There are also an escalating number of cohesive efforts to shape the responses of the government, health insurers, and mainstream medicine, as well as the behavior of the public, particularly persons with defined health care needs. The totality of these efforts is best understood as the beginning of a convergence between the occupations and professions that comprise alternative medicine. But many questions remain. To what degree does "alternative medicine" comprise a category with which people identify? Do people who use the techniques that we've called "alternative medicine" see themselves as consumers or practitioners of alternative medicine? Or do they consider what they are doing to be *solely* or primarily within some other, more limited, domain such as "homeopathy," "chelation therapy," or "herbal medicine"? Do "insiders" identify alternative medicine as a coherent phenomenon by what they say (or write) about it, and how they behave toward it?

It is easy to find alternative practitioners representing many different therapeutic approaches who explicitly situate their work within a broader category of "alternative" or "holistic" medicine. James Gordon, a psychiatrist and well known practitioner of "integral medicine," reports on practitioners of psychic healing, biofeedback, meditation, chiropractic, herbal medicine, TCM, homeopathy, and many other forms of healing who agree that their own work falls within a "holistic paradigm." More recent compendia, such as the thousand-plus page *Alternative Medicine: The Definitive Guide,* bring together a vast array of approaches to healing as self-consciously subscribing to "a common philosophy that: focuses on empowering the individual to accept responsibility for at least part of the task of recovery . . . recommends a balanced lifestyle . . . and emotional tranquility . . . recognizes the importance of . . . the body's energy pathways. . . [and] . . . most importantly, treats the individual instead of his or her symptoms." A similar volume, *Alternative Healing: The Complete A–Z Guide to More Than 150 Alternative Therapies,* emphasizes that for each intervention "the basic philosophy is the same. . . . Alternative medicine treats people, not just their diseases . . . treats causes rather than symptoms . . . is interested in maintaining good health through the prevention of disease . . . and understands that there is a crucial relationship between body, mind, and spirit." There is a great deal of published material for both consumers and practitioners that depicts alternative medicine as a cohesive, "real" phenomenon.

Of course, it is not surprising to find that volumes which explicitly market themselves as being about alternative medicine support the notion that such a thing exists. Still, the growing number of such works and the extent of their sales indicate that there are practitioners who do see alternative medicine as a distinct entity, and that a portion of the public is responsive to this categorization.

It is more telling to examine how practitioners of particular types of therapy situate their approaches relative to a broader category like alternative or holistic medicine. The attitudes of practitioners of the older, more well established healing systems are quite mixed, ranging from very low to very high identification with a broad classification of alternative medicine. But it is fair to say that these individuals are beginning at least to partially identify with alternative medicine, although they may prefer to use the terms "complementary" or "holistic" medicine.

An excellent example of this growing affiliation or identification with alternative medicine can be found in the writing of Deepak Chopra. Chopra is an Indian-born physician who trained and practiced endocrinology in the United States. Through his contact with Maharishi Mahesh Yogi (best known for bringing Transcendental Meditation to the United States), Chopra turned back to the practice of Ayurvedic medicine, eventually becoming its most well-known American popularizer and exponent. His books have sold many millions of copies. Through these volumes and his videotapes, audiotapes, lectures and seminars, Chopra has become one of the best known exponents of alternative medicine in the country, and by far the single most well-established advocate of Ayurvedic medicine. It is useful to look at how his writing over the past few years has evolved.

Chopra's two largest selling volumes are *Quantum Healing* and *Ageless Body, Timeless Mind*. While both books cover a similar range of topics, Ayurvedic medicine merits sixteen page references in the index of the earlier volume, as opposed to only one in the more recent work. The first book, dedicated to the Maharishi, openly presents itself as an attempt to introduce Ayurvedic medicine to a Western audience: "I needed to show that this was a science in its own right. How to do that? It would come. Indian thought has always been grounded on the conviction that *Satya,* the truth, alone triumphs. 'The truth is simple,' Maharishi encouraged. 'Make it clear, let it stand on its own, and don't get lost in complications.'" In *Quantum Healing,* Chopra explicitly states that among the holistic approaches to healing, Ayurvedic medicine is "better than any alternative, although it may not be very apparent on the surface," and he claims that Ayurvedic medicine is the basis of TCM. In contrast, *Ageless Body, Timeless Mind* is grounded in references to Western mind-body medicine, psychoneuroimmunology, and physics. Ayurvedic medicine is not even defined for the reader until the last quarter of the book.

Both of Chopra's books effectively and articulately advocate a range of preventive and healing techniques built upon mobilizing the body, especially the immune system, through meditation, imagery, and lifestyle change. The earlier book (*Quantum Healing*) is clear that the three most important techniques emerge from what Ayurveda calls "bliss." "Ayurveda has made use of this principle for thousands of years. Indeed, since the basic premise of Vedic knowledge is that consciousness creates the body, it is only natural that techniques for focusing attention should have been discovered. . . . The bliss techniques . . . fall into this category." The same techniques are presented in *Ageless Body, Timeless Mind* (published in 1993), but their origin in Ayurvedic "bliss" is not so clearly stated. When the reader is told near the end of the book that in order for your efforts to succeed you should "Follow your bliss," the quote is attributed to the mythologist Joseph Campbell. When the 1993 volume speaks of "chi," the life force in TCM, it simply notes that this notion exists in Ayurveda as Prana, as it does in Sufism, Christianity, and "many cultural traditions." The newer book's purpose is not to carry the word of the Maharishi, but to teach us about "a new paradigm" where awareness is "the fundamental stuff of life. In all religious traditions the breath of life is spirit." Looking at Chopra's writing over time, it is clear that he has shifted his tone. The specific Ayurvedic tradition is relatively less emphasized, replaced by a broader acceptance of other healing traditions and techniques. His is one prominent example of a practitioner of a specific modality who has begun to promote "alternative medicine" as a cohesive reality.

In March of 1995 a new journal, *Alternative Therapies,* began publication as a "forum for sharing information concerning the practical use of alternative therapies in preventing and treating disease, healing illness, and promoting health." *Alternative Therapies* "does not endorse any particular methodology, but promotes the evaluation and appropriate use of all effective approaches from the physical to the transpersonal." Well known advocates of every major approach to alternative healing appear on the advisory and editorial boards, as well as among the authors. The editor, Larry Dossey, writes that the mission of the journal is "to encourage the development of a lingua franca, a common language. . . . In doing so we hope to calm the acrimony that too often substitutes for calm debate in this field."

A desire for a "lingua franca" is becoming a real part of the professional lives of many alternative practitioners. The creation and acceptance of a common set of symbols/vocabulary is a good measure of whether or not alternative medicine exists as a true entity. While this goal has yet to be fully realized, it is evident that movement toward it is underway. To the extent that an allegiance to a common set of core beliefs is reflected by the use of a common language, alternative medicine would appear to be an increasingly cohesive phenomenon.

Alternative Medicine as a Professional Entity

Professions are usually characterized as those occupations that have achieved the greatest degree of autonomy over their work. One group is more professional than another based upon its ability to decide what, how, and when work needs to be done, as well as upon its power to evaluate whether or not the work has been done well. The attainment of high professional power and status is due to the concerted efforts of elite elements within an occupation who make professionalization a goal. Successful attempts to professionalize require the development of professional organizations, educational standards, credentials, a sense of cohesiveness, and most of all an acceptance by other political and economic elites within a society. Becoming a profession is a long-term and ongoing process, success is a matter of degree, and the potential to become more or less "professional" is always present. To what extent does alternative medicine have the characteristics that constitute a profession?

Twenty-five years ago, there were no organized groupings of "alternative," "holistic" or "complementary" health care providers in the United States. Instead, there were organizations comprised solely of chiropractors, osteopaths, and a few other types of non-mainstream health care providers. Today the situation is far different. A number of organizations and associations exist that encompass multiple alternative practices. They espouse a wide array of aims that include continuing education, disseminating information, conducting research, gaining recognition from the state via licensure, the direct provision of services and care, and mutual support of like-minded practitioners. The organizations vary considerably in terms of how restrictive their entrance requirements are, as well as how they approach various issues in the field. Goals within and between organizations frequently conflict on matters such as who is deserving of professional credentials, the advantages of limited professional acceptance under the supervision of M.D.'s, and the proper role of certain modes of care. At the same time, the number of organizations devoted to furthering the work and professional status of particular specialties, such as acupuncture, reflexology, naturopathy, or massage therapy, have also mushroomed. Some, among the hundreds of such organizations, work toward the singular advancement of a particular group, while others advocate for more inclusive recognition of other alternative approaches along with their own. Thus, the situation is complex and fluid.

Despite the ambiguity, alternative medicine has a considerably greater organizational reality than ever before. An overriding goal of these groups is to foster an approach that includes multiple techniques of care among the general public, the government, and the world of mainstream medicine. For example, the American Holistic Medical Association (AHMA) is a group of about six hundred physicians and medical students whose goal is "to support physicians in their evolving personal and professional development and to promote an art and science of health care which acknowledges all aspects of the individual, the family and the planet." Although full membership is restricted to current and future M.D.'s, the organization is open to those who practice many specific forms of care from naturopathy to homeopathy, Ayurvedic medicine, and TCM. Associate membership is available to "all state licensed, holistically oriented practitioners, such as chiropractors, naturopaths, nurses, psychologists, dentists, etc." A similar group is the four thousand-member American Holistic Nurses Association (AHNA), founded in 1980 "by a group of nurses dedicated to bringing the concepts of holism to every area of nursing practice." The mission of the AHNA is to "create opportunities for nurses to heal and empower ourselves and others through modeling and integrating holism in our lives and practices." Both the AHMA and the AHNA give their members opportunities for continuing medical education courses (and credits), mutual social support, and practical advice on integrating holistic techniques and styles into the mainstream professions.

At the other end of the continuum are groups like PATH, the Professional Association of Traditional Healers, which has no restrictions on who may belong. Its aim is "bringing together all traditions of healing . . . to promote collaboration, integration, and bridging. . . ." Another organization, the American Association for Holistic Health, was formed to serve "all who are interested in holistic health and wellness, particularly in regard to the combined utilization of both traditional and alternative medicine." This all-inclusive group promotes itself as a national- and state-level lobbying organization and information clearinghouse.

Scores of similar groups have come into existence over the past decade. Although most don't survive very long, some do. Many of the larger and more successful groups develop educational or training programs for both alternative health providers and mainstream health professionals. Typical is a symposium on alternative medicine organized in 1995 by the International Spa and Fitness Association with the cooperation of the National Institutes of Health. Billed as an educational seminar for health and fitness professionals of all backgrounds, the day-long meeting offered sessions on "spontaneous healing," "touch therapy," "the power of prayer," and "relaxation response and healing" as well as talks on integrating different natural healing modalities into mainstream care.

Much more elaborate and lengthy courses are now widespread. Many of these programs have professional organizations, publications, and educational institutions as co-sponsors. One of the most successful is the series created by the journal *Alternative Therapies* and the University of Arizona School of Medicine. Like the journal, these sessions do not endorse any particular form of healing, and have included practitioners representing at least a dozen major alternative approaches. Similar courses have been sponsored by Harvard's School of Medicine (jointly with the School's Mind-Body Medical Institute) and scores of other highly regarded medical schools. The goals of Harvard's annual courses on "Spirituality and Healing," were to explore "the relationship between spirituality and healing in medicine from the perspective of major world religions" and to provide participants with an understanding of "the scientific evidence for the effects of spirituality on healing, the physiological and neurologic effects of healing resulting from spirituality, and the relationship amongst healing, spirituality, and mind/body effects." The courses, each of which has been attended by over 900 mainstream practitioners, have offered presentations by a wide array of advocates for different approaches to healing, religion, and spirituality.

Clearly, a number of organizations exist whose goal is to present alternative medicine as a coherent and cohesive entity to the public. Some are profit making, and others are nonprofit. But all of them take an inclusive view of alternative medicine, and many are explicit about grounding their practices in the underlying beliefs and assumptions of the alternative worldview.

In many larger cities and regions, the creation of alternative medicine directories along with referral services, fairs, and "health expos" has become a large enterprise. "Whole Life Expo," which began in Pasadena in 1982 and now holds "expos" in six cities (San Francisco, San Jose, Minneapolis, Austin, Chicago, Atlanta) on a regular basis, is typical of these operations. The programs at such events include much in addition to alternative medicine: spirituality, art, music, and various forms of "new age" motivational speakers are all heavily represented. The Omega Institute for Holistic Studies in Rhinebeck, New York, is one of a number of organizations that offers a more upscale set of seminars in major cities around the country through the year and on its campus during the spring and summer. The subjects range from month-long intensive training in movement therapy, yoga, and massage ($2,300), through "wellness weeks" ($320) and introductory weekend retreats ($120–$350) on topics like "Unintentional Healing"; "The Shamanic Journey, Power and Healing"; "Nutritional Therapy in Medical Practice"; "The Dance of Tennis"; "Medicine Teachings of the Earth: Northwest Coast and Native American Shamanism"; "Iyengar Yoga for Practicing, Teaching and Sharing"; and "Healing Hands: Using the Human Energy Field." These courses contain a dual focus on health and wellness instruction for individuals and training for professionals. The great majority of their presentations are grounded in a commitment to the core beliefs of an alternative worldview. The professional training programs include weekend-long workshops in a wide variety of alternative modalities, including nutritional therapy, massage therapy, reflexology, mindfulness-based stress reduction, past life therapy, hypnosis, and holistic nursing.

Alternative Therapies itself is a good example of how far efforts to create an inclusive professional identity have gone. The journal offers "a forum for sharing information. . . . [It] does not endorse any particular methodology, but promotes the evaluation and appropriate use of all effective approaches from the physical to the transpersonal . . . [and] publishes . . . high quality scientific research. The journal encourages the integration of alternative therapies with conventional medical practices in a way that provides for a rational, individualized, comprehensive approach to health care." A second journal with a similar mandate, *The Journal of Alternative and Complementary Medicine,* has also recently begun to publish "high quality" scientific research articles on a wide range of therapies. The creation of these periodicals is a clear effort to provide a foundation for the professional status of alternative medicine.

Many groups of alternative providers around the nation have created more substantial training programs to give practitioners of one specific mode of care some experience beyond their primary disciplinary training. A typical example is the California Institute of Integral Studies in San Francisco, which among its many courses and degree programs offers degrees and certificates in "integral health studies" for those who already are trained in some aspect of health care. It claims to provide "added qualifications" for such people by teaching them to apply the "pluralistic, holistic and ecological framework of integral health"; "build bridges between Eastern, Western and Indigenous healing systems; acknowledge the mental, emotional, and spiritual realms beyond the physical body; apply the feminine principle to the underlying medical paradigm; explore applications of new paradigms in science to health and healing; and affirm the deep connection between human and global ecology." The Program in Integrative Medicine, under the direction of Dr. Andrew Weil at the University of Arizona, offers "a variety of professional development and CME [continuing medical education] activities designed to meet the needs of physicians and professional health care providers in clinical practice" including "a quarterly mini-conference series [that] introduces topics in integrative medicine" and "comprehensive conferences focusing on integrative medicine for various specialty areas." The Program in Integrative Medicine also offers a two-year fellowship for physicians (M.D. or D.O.) who have completed residencies in primary care specialties: "The goal of this innovative program is to train fellows in healing oriented, safe, and effective treatments that combine the best ideas and practices of conventional and alternative medicine." The curriculum at the University of Arizona includes training in a variety of healing modalities, including mind/body medicine, nutritional medicine, botanical medicine, energy medicine, interactive guided imagery, medical acupuncture, homeopathy, and osteopathic manipulative therapy, and is oriented towards "doctors, nurses, pharmacists, medical students, and physicians in practice." In both their openness to many types of healers and in their willingness to educate participants about many types of modalities, these programs intend to create a common body of knowledge and professional identity for alternative practitioners.

Research institutes with the goal of clinically evaluating the full range of alternative approaches using standard research methods have also begun to emerge. The Complete Wellness Research Institute, under the direction of Marc

Micozzi, M.D., Ph.D., wants its "seal of approval" to be the gold standard for alternative treatments. Micozzi, a pathologist and former senior investigator at the National Cancer Institute, was the founding director of the National Museum of Health and Medicine. His idea for the Complete Wellness Research Institute and the Complete Wellness Medical Centers (a national network of clinics where the products and techniques holding the "seal of approval" would be offered) emerged after he assembled and edited a well-received text for alternative practitioners and students. His work is one of a number of similar efforts currently underway to establish a well-defined professional identity for alternative providers.

Gaining Legal Acceptance

Recognition and acceptance by the government through legislation and administrative fiat is a key indicator of a group's recognition and acceptance by the larger society. In the 1980s, Jack Salmon and Howard Berliner described a number of policy considerations raised by "the holistic health movement." The issues included gaining third-party reimbursement, creating licensure and certification for alternative practitioners, integrating into mainstream medical settings, and obtaining funding for research on the efficacy of alternative therapies and for holistic health centers. The authors recognized that in each case the government would play a crucial role in fostering or inhibiting such changes. In 1980 the discussion was purely conceptual and hypothetical, as the movement was in "such a nebulous and eclectic" state. Since 1980, however, there has been significant government involvement in each of these areas, indicating that alternative medicine has come far as an ongoing entity in the world. For the most part, these developments have benefited alternative therapy as a whole, instead of merely legitimizing specific techniques.

In a report commissioned by the Fetzer Institute, David Sale provided the best summary description of governmental action with regard to alternative medicine. The amount of change since Salmon and Berliner set out their speculations fifteen years earlier is impressive. Besides chiropractic and osteopathy, which are recognized in all states, there are provider practice acts for acupuncture (twenty-six states and the District of Columbia), homeopathy (three states), massage therapy (twenty jurisdictions with statewide recognition in eight states), and naturopathy (nine states). In most instances, states specifically extend the right to practice these better known forms of care to encompass a number of other alternative modalities. Thus, "the scope of practice for naturopathy includes such well known alternative modalities as acupuncture, biofeedback, homeopathy, hypnotherapy, or massage." Some states even include minor surgery in this list. Twenty-seven other specific types of alternative therapy have received limited recognition by the states. The states of Alaska, Washington, North Carolina, South Dakota, New York, and Maryland (as well as Arizona subsequent to Sale's report) have expanded their medical practice acts to specify the right of conventional physicians to practice alternative therapies without incurring professional sanctions. Although these state laws are each somewhat distinct, they generally recognize that alternative therapies as a whole, rather than any specific modality, deserve protection. Sale repeatedly notes the "convergence" of many forms of alternative therapy in every type of legislation, whether written from the standpoint of the consumer who wishes access to them or providers who seek the right to use them in their practice. He writes, "This legislative pattern suggests the existence of a multidisciplinary orientation and fluidity in practice boundaries for many alternative providers that may not be matched among allopathic providers."

On the national level almost all legislative and regulatory activity has treated alternative therapies as a whole, rather than singling out specific modes of care. The most notable example is the founding of The Office of Alternative Medicine, whose very name is indicative of the trend. The legislation establishing OAM (discussed at greater length in Chapter 6) not only offers proof of federal recognition of alternative medicine as an entity deserving of the government's protection and funds, but also offers a powerful symbolic message as well. Speaking about OAM, David Hufford notes: "If they cannot gain public acceptance, knowledge claims and assertions of authority remain only that—claims and assertions. Public acceptance of legitimacy is complete only when it has become habitual. . . . That is why the struggle always involves language. . . . In the 1960s the language of health in the United States began to alter. . . . In 1970 there was no common English term to aggregate 'alternative medicine.'" The decision to include "alternative medicine" in the name of the official federal agency reflects the growing acceptance of the term and reinforces it by bestowing even more legitimacy upon it. Over a period when cutbacks in federal funding have been the norm, the amount of money allocated for OAM has steadily grown. OAM's budget authorization by Congress increased six-fold, from $2 million to $12 million between 1992 and 1997.

Much of OAM's activities over the first few years of its life (1992–1996) have been directed toward establishing the field of alternative medicine as a legitimate entity. The various conferences, publications, advisory boards, newsletters, and funding priorities that emerged from the agency have brought together advocates of many different modes of care. Thus, the agency's first round of thirty research grants went to study over twenty different treatment modalities. Only massage (four), guided imagery (four), acupuncture (two), and Ayurvedic medicine (two) received more than a single grant. A second set of twelve awards was more focused, with half the grants going to study various aspects of TCM. OAM's first two grants for the establishment of centers ($840,000 each) went to institutions that were attempting to study a variety of alternative treatments for a single problem (for example, HIV/AIDS and addictive disorders). An ongoing OAM goal has been to bring together researchers and practitioners from different areas, especially for the purpose of developing a set of common research criteria and methods.

Recognition by Conventional Medicine

The relationship between alternative and conventional medicine is complex. Until recently, the dominant view within the mainstream medical institutions and professional associations has been that the vast array of alternative techniques and approaches are a singular phenomenon, albeit unified by their unscientific status and often equated with quackery. The following quote is from the Proceedings of the 1973 AMA House of Delegates Meeting:

> [There is] the need to root out the nonscientific substitutes with rational medical care. The fakes, the frauds, and the quackeries need to be identified, exposed, and, if possible, eradicated. This is not an easy task. A gullible public is all too easily entranced with food faddism and pseudoscientific diets. Legislators have been all too willing to incorporate chiropractic benefits into federal and state health care programs. Uncontrolled acupuncture has been legalized in at least one jurisdiction. Yet where individuals have been able to do little, the AMA has acted effectively in helping to put an end to Hoxsey-type promotions, to expose Krebiozen, and on and on and on. It is plainly contrary to the public interest to permit the development of new kinds of health professionals without supervision and controls. On the one hand, it seems possible to educate and train men and women to fill immensely useful roles in supplementation of, and extension to, the work of physicians. On the other hand, there is the possibility that new kinds of pseudo-professionals, ill-trained and uncontrolled, might turn the clock back to the pre-Flexner-AMA days of diploma mills and dubious credentials.

As recently as 1993, in a guidebook for consumers published by the AMA, alternative methods are defined as "unproven, disproven, controversial, fraudulent, quack, and/or otherwise questionable approaches to solving health problems." In 1997, Arnold Relman, the esteemed past editor of the *New England Journal of Medicine,* described Andrew Weil's work this way: "Throughout history people have wanted to believe that there are easy, natural ways to defeat disease, and there have always been people like Andrew Weil who peddle a variety of snake oil." Late that same year, Dr. Wallace Sampson, a clinical professor of medicine at Stanford and long-time critic of alternative medicine, launched a new journal, *The Scientific Review of Alternative Medicine,* with the expressed goal of subjecting alternative therapies to skeptical analysis. The journal's publisher is Paul Kurtz, who chairs the Committee for the Scientific Investigation of Claims of the Paranormal and has the backing of a group of outspoken physician critics of alternative medicine that calls itself the Council for Scientific Medicine. The journal's first issue found homeopathy, chelation therapy, therapeutic touch, and the writings of Andrew Weil all lacking support. Yet, mainstream medicine is beginning to move beyond this longstanding hostile view.

Conventional medicine's recognition of alternative forms of care has largely consisted of piecemeal utilization of particular therapies, such as biofeedback for hypertension or guided imagery to reduce chronic pain. For the most part, this acceptance has been scattered and hesitant. *Time* magazine included a section on alternative medicine in a special issue on the "frontiers of medicine." But it framed the discussion by asking, "The big question remains: Does all this newfound Establishment attention mean that the nonconventional therapies really work?" Increasingly, mainstream physicians' answer is "we don't know, but maybe, and we'd like to know more." Surveys of internists and other primary care doctors have found that, on average, they perceive acupuncture and manipulations as "moderately effective" and a much longer list (diet, biofeed-back, massage, hypnotherapy, etc.) as "legitimate," if unproven, medical interventions. What puts off those doctors is their inability to understand why such treatments are effective.

The issue was clearly articulated by Senator Tom Harkin of Iowa, who was one of the most influential politicians in the establishment and ongoing funding of the OAM. His statement to the alternative community was clear: "Mainstreaming alternative practices that work is our next step." But he immediately added, "One challenge in bridging the gap . . . is defining the terms by which we find each others methodology acceptable and efficacious. . . . Keep in mind that it was not too long ago . . . we could not see germs and therefore could not accept their existence. Could there be something we are not 'seeing' here that is key to these therapies? . . . We must find an approach where the unbendable rules of randomized clinical trials and the uncertainty of anecdotal case studies are laid aside in favor of a third approach—one that will quantify the effectiveness of therapies without breaking them down into a series of chemical reactions and physiological processes. . . . It is not necessary for the scientific community to understand the process before the American people can benefit from these therapies." In other words, there needs to be an acceptance of the broader paradigm of alternative care, along with the recognition of specific forms of clinical efficacy.

Conventional providers recognize alternative medicine as a comprehensive approach or set of assumptions much less frequently. Still, such recognition is growing. Dean Ornish's Preventive Medicine Research Institute in San Francisco has become widely recognized for its use of a fundamentally alternative perspective along with many specific forms of alternative care in reversing the course of cardiovascular disease. Under the leadership of Ron Anderson, Parkland Hospital in Dallas has tried to apply the principles of mind/body medicine throughout the institution and the community. These two examples are often cited as models of mainstream care that incorporates alternative medicine principles. More recently, Columbia Presbyterian Medical Center and the Columbia College of Physicians and Surgeons opened The Richard and Hilda Rosenthal Center for Complementary and Alternative Medicine and The Center for Complementary and Alternative Medicine Research in Women's Health. Both centers sponsor research projects, alternative medicine grand rounds series, and symposia on various topics in alternative medicine. The NIH provides funding to centers for research on alternative medicine at the University of Virginia, the Kessler Institute for Rehabilitation, Columbia University, the University of Texas, Harvard Medical School, the Minneapolis Medical Research Center, Bastyr University, UC Davis, and Stanford University as well as the Palmer College of Chiropractic. All of these medical schools are among the seventy-five that now include courses on complementary and alternative medicine in their curricula. Little is known about how many students enroll, the actual content of the courses, or how that content is related to the broader educational experience. There are a growing number of clinics—such as the Spence Clinic for Women in Massachusetts, the American Holistic Centers in the Midwest, and the Arizona Center for Health and Medicine in Phoenix—that utilize a holistic or alternative approach alongside conventional care. These facilities claim a great deal of success in terms of client satisfaction, reduced costs, and therapeutic benefits. Yet the rise of these profit-making facilities does not signify the same degree of acceptance by mainstream medicine as do the university-based medical centers.

Another indication of the growing acceptance of alternative medicine is the decision of Oxford Health Plan to add alternative medicine coverage to some of its health plans. While other health insurance companies—such as American Western Life Insurance, Blue Cross, and Kaiser Permanente—also provide limited coverage for alternative medical services, Oxford Health Plan was the first major insurance company to establish a full plan. Oxford provides care to 1.4 million people in the eastern United States and will make alternative care available to its members in New York, New Jersey, and Connecticut. The initial network of alternative providers includes "about 1,000 chiropractors, acupuncturists, naturopaths, massage therapists and yoga instructors," and the addition of practitioners of T'ai Chi and reflexology is anticipated. The chief executive of Oxford said "that the company considered alternative medicine an addition to traditional care, not a replacement," and that Oxford will study whether the use of alternative care improves patient's health or affects cost.

Individual professionals with interests in alternative medicine have had some success in getting mainstream organizations to include their concerns. Groups such as the American Society of Clinical Oncology have offered sessions on spirituality and cancer survival at their annual meetings. In 1997, the American Cancer Society decided to "soften its terminology" when referring to nontraditional approaches to cancer treatment: "In the past, the ACS had referred to such treatments as 'questionable'; however, in light of changing attitudes about complementary therapies, the ACS now refers to such practices as 'alternative and complementary.'" In 1993, the American Public Health Association created a "special primary interest group" within the organization for those members concerned with "Alternative and Complementary Health Services." Two years later, the American Medical Association passed a resolution suggesting that its three hundred thousand members "become better informed regarding the practices and techniques of alternative and unconventional medicine." Organizations concerned with medical ethics, such as the Hastings Center and The Park Ridge Center, have begun to discuss the implications of an alternative point of view.

Despite the sort of developments just mentioned, the acceptance of alternative perspectives by the medical mainstream is still a highly tentative and contentious process. As mentioned before, the new journal the *Scientific Review of Alternative Medicine* openly holds that its goal is debunking alternative medicine. The editor, Dr. Wallace Sampson, says that "alternative" and "complementary" are euphemisms for "it doesn't work." In mid-1998, *JAMA* published an article attacking the validity of "therapeutic touch" that has over forty-seven thousand practitioners, consisting mostly of R.N.'s. A nine-year-old girl had done the research as a project for a school science fair. As the research did not involve anyone with a disorder that therapeutic touch claims to treat and the girl had been assisted by her mother, an outspoken critic of therapeutic touch, as well as two national leaders of anti-alternative medicine organizations, the work was hardly unbiased.

Bonnie Blair O'Connor's descriptive research on the use of alternative therapies to treat AIDS is one of the best accounts of the complexities in the ongoing relationship of alternative and conventional medicine. People with AIDS have tried a lengthy list of alternative therapies including herbal preparations, vitamin supplements, physical manipulation, and homeopathy to halt the progression of HIV into AIDS. Dozens of other techniques are frequently used expressly to moderate symptoms and side effects of conventional drugs and other therapies. A major goal of those who are HIV positive is to maintain the strength of their immune system. As many forms of alternative medicine are oriented toward strengthening the immune system and conventional medicine has little to offer in this regard, one might expect Western doctors to be more receptive to alternative forms of care. Yet, as O'Connor relates, this has generally not occurred. Thus, even for a problem where conventional treatment has had little to offer and where alternative care is well established, acceptance by the mainstream has been limited. On the other hand, in 1996 a panel of "114 leading scientists and representatives of academia, drug companies, community organizations, and AIDS advocates" urged the National Institutes of Health "to strengthen the scientific base to determine the safety and effectiveness of alternative medicine research therapies for AIDS." In recommending that the NIH invest in research on "alternative medicine" rather than any specific modality, the wording of the panel indicates that the mainstream is beginning to recognize alternative medicine as a cohesive phenomena.

Overall, mainstream medicine has historically not accepted the idea of alternative medicine as a cohesive entity. Rather, most recognition has come in terms of limited therapeutic interventions. However, this seems to be changing, fostered and heightened by the overall economic and organizational forces influencing conventional care.

The Mass Media and the Public

The general public is increasingly familiar and comfortable with the term "alternative medicine." That phrase, and other inclusive names such as "holistic medicine" and "complementary medicine" frequently appear in the mass media. When these terms come up, there is typically some explicit or implicit recognition that the various techniques included are linked by a common set of assumptions and beliefs. In *Time* magazine's special issue on "The Frontiers of Medicine" in the Fall of 1996, acupuncture, biofeedback, chiropractic, homeopathy, and other unconventional techniques were described as "alternative" medicine in part because they all emphasize "human contact" in their relations with clients. Similarly, a *New York Times Magazine* article on people with cancer grouped techniques such as acupuncture, yoga, prayer groups, and megavitamins all together as "alternative" therapies. The major conclusion of the piece, as well as the implicit justification for considering these various techniques together, was an affirmation of one of alternative medicine's core beliefs: for a therapy to be effective, it must make sense to the individual. Clearly, over the past several years, the media increasingly has been using the phrase "alternative medicine" to represent a coherent system of beliefs.

An important source of information about nonconventional forms of health care for the public are magazines like *New Age Journal*, *Prevention*, and *Natural Healing*, all of which view alternative medicine as an inclusive, coherent phenomenon. These are widely read publications. *Prevention* estimates that its total average paid circulation is 3,311,224 and that each copy is read by 3.41 persons, indicating a total audience of more than eleven million people. *New Age Journal* estimates its readership at a quarter of a million. Illustrating the orientation of these magazines is the "Holistic Health Directory" published by *New Age Journal*, which encompasses more than six thousand practitioners of about one hundred forty different approaches. The body of the directory is preceded by a series of articles (including one co-authored by former First Lady Rosalynn Carter) educating readers about alternative approaches to care and how to select the specific treatment and practitioner best for them. Locally produced directories of alternative practitioners can now be found in most every area of the country. A typical example from the San Juan Islands in Washington State has listings for about forty different types of healers. Interspersed are descriptions of the techniques, and the preface "Why Alternative Medicine?" specifies that the healers are included in the directory based upon their common practice of four key principles: vitalism, integration of body-mind-spirit, individualized treatment, and emphasis on the healing process.

Most recently, the Internet and the World Wide Web have become important sources of information about alternative medicine. Although websites on most every imaginable aspect of alternative care are accessible, the most widely used are those that offer a comprehensive and inclusive approach. Sites such as "Ask Dr. Weil" and the "Alternative Medicine Homepage" recognize the commonalties between the range of alternative approaches and offer those who log on the opportunity to link up with a vast array of more specific resources. Similar to the magazines, institutes, and other organizations that promote alternative therapies, these sites consciously bring many different types of techniques together to represent a broader understanding of health and healing. For example, the Alternative Health and Healing Forum (a newsgroup of America Online) offers interactive programs on alternative HIV/AIDS care, hypnosis, biofeedback, yoga, and nutrition. According to Dr. Dan Casper, the forum's "content coordinator," the intention of the forum is to provide "usable, understandable, and accurate information on available alternative therapies." On the Web, the Alchemical Medicine Research and Teaching Association (AMRTA) provides nationwide listings of upcoming conferences, symposia, and lectures covering an almost staggering number of modalities and topics: homeopathy, acupuncture, lucid dreaming, thought field therapy, mindfulness-based stress reduction, herbal medicine, spirituality and healing, integrative medicine, altered states and shamanistic practice, etc. Even sites that are hostile, like "Quackwatch," offer a critical stance toward many alternative approaches because of what they have in common, such as a belief in vitalism.

This growing convergence around the phrase "alternative medicine" and the acceptance of its underlying assumptions does not mean that specific therapeutic approaches have halted their own efforts to promote themselves, establish publications, or gain certification. All the most well known modes of care, such as homeopathy, chiropractic, and many, many others have continued or even increased their efforts. However, we can view even these more focused concerns as taking place within a broader context of alternative medicine. Thus, readers of the

Yoga Journal will find favorable references to many other alternative medicine Internet sites in its "Webwatch" section, along with laudatory reports on developments outside of yoga, such as the decision by OAM to fund a natural medicine clinic in Seattle that will use a wide range of conventional and alternative approaches. A lead editorial in *Homeopathy Today,* a journal for practicing homeopaths, condemns an attack on "alternative health care" by noting that the essence of homeopathy is "a continuation of the vitalistic and empirical tradition in western medicine" and emphasizes how developments in quantum physics and chaos theory are validating a nonmechanistic view of reality. A promotional pamphlet from the Foot Reflexology Awareness Association promises that membership will bring education and training about reflexology "and other holistic ways to health and well-being." These are each typical examples of the growing trend of specific nonconventional modes of care to utilize mass media to identify themselves as part of a broader entity: alternative medicine.

Alternative Medicine as an Identity

Much about alternative medicine's growing cohesiveness still has a vague and superficial quality, however. Definitions of basic terms, certification procedures, standards of care, and measures of outcomes are all in their infancy, frequently contested, and held in disrepute by many. Much of what exists is held together by a largely pragmatic entrepreneurial ethos and the common bond of being "outsiders."

What makes "alternative medicine" a useful phrase is not its ability to define a clear-cut world of organizations and procedures. Rather, the cohesion represented by the phrase centers around a system of meaning with which a growing number of people are identifying. It is an identity based in part on a shared set of understandings about what is missing from the dominant medical understanding of health and illness. As a political or organizational phenomenon, alternative medicine is in its infancy. But, as an aspect of our culture that can offer a cohesive collective identity, it is entering its adolescence.

According to social psychologists, collective identity is built "through shared definitions of the situation" through an "ongoing process of interaction, negotiation, and conflict"; it is "a moving target, with different definitions predominating at different points." A collective identity is cognitively real, if organizationally and substantively messy. The very ambiguity and partly formed nature of alternative medicine allows many groups and practitioners to identify with it. It is not necessary to give up any other identities one may possess. Someone can remain a physician, or an acupuncturist, or simply a sufferer of a chronic illness and at the same time identify with alternative medicine. Indeed, it may be preferable to combine alternative medicine with another identity (or identities) if this facilitates a personal or professional transformation. In the same way that feminism is an additive and transformative identity (as when one self identifies as a "feminist historian"), one can be an "alternative physician" or a "person with cancer who is into alternative medicine." Such identities connote, at a minimum, a critical stance toward conventional practices and an openness toward the core assumptions of the alternative worldview.

Sociologists are now recognizing that a social movement can exist primarily in the form of "meaning" as opposed to a collection of organizations with clearly articulated and coordinated goals. As in the case of the feminist movement, or the civil rights or gay liberation movements, individuals may be deeply affected and feel they "belong" to the movement for many years while never having any organizational affiliation. The structural dimension of the movement exists, but it is highly fluid, and of secondary importance, compared to the sense of identity the movement offers and the options it presents for social change.

Joseph Gusfield has claimed that "in one sense, a social movement exists when members of a society share the recognition that specific rules are no longer taken for granted." As an example of one of these "new" noninstitutional social movements, he cites "holistic health. . . . Here there is no organizational base at all. The dissidence is not directed at changing the state or an institution. . . . They are dissenting movements within medicine, but they do little to change professional medicine, develop new state laws, or protest current medical or hospital practice." For Gusfield, the ideas and identities of the holistic health movement are enough to create its reality. While the ideological or ideational reality he refers to is strong and growing, the institutional and organizational structure of alternative medicine, which he dismisses, is far from absent.

Many organizations exist primarily to "spread the word" about the core beliefs and assumptions of the alternative worldview to the general public and other health care providers. Aspects of these efforts can almost take on the quality of a moral crusade. The names of the books (*Back to Eden, Between Heaven and Earth*), programs ("Earth as Utopia" at the Omega Institute) and clinics (*Avalon* Health Associates in Worcester, Massachusetts) often have a utopian quality about them. The message that they give, and the identity they offer, is that the misfortune of illness is not inevitable. Just reading or buying a book whose title is *Total Health* or *Ageless Body, Timeless Mind* implies something about what one believes might be possible and thus affirms an identity distinct from the conventional view. These books, seminars, and websites provide an institutional basis for expressing a "critical distance" from conventional scientific medicine and asserting the possibility of transformation for both oneself and the society. The growing number of alternative medical institutions provides a concrete means of resisting the dominant form of medical knowledge by pointing out its inconsistencies and paradoxes, as well as by providing examples of things that happen which the dominant view says cannot.

These institutional manifestations of alternative medicine are not important merely because they conform to a traditional view of social movements that seeks organizational coherence and stability. In an "information-based society," their ability to provide an ongoing flow of fact, opinion, and symbols is crucial. Much of the information that is offered by the institutionalized organs of alternative medicine is detailed and highly specific: what to eat, how to treat a symptom, etc. But often this information is placed within the broader context of a moral crusade for a deeper and more fundamental change in basic values and assumptions. It is in terms of conceptual values and beliefs that alternative medicine's diverse tapestry (or cacophony) of systems and techniques can find a common sense of identity.

Freedom and Health

The common identity offered by alternative medicine is based largely upon the shared core beliefs described in the preceding chapters. But as another aspect of their shared identity, and to justify their recognition and legitimacy in the larger society, alternative practitioners and institutions consistently attach themselves to the deeply rooted American value of personal freedom.

Freedom is perhaps the most cherished ideal in the American belief system. The War of Independence, Bill of Rights, Civil War, and countless other historical events, documents and symbols in American history derive their meaning and currency from the identity of the United States as "the home of the free." The freedom to believe what one wishes and to act upon those beliefs, insofar as it doesn't hurt someone else, is highly cherished. Freedom to associate with like-minded individuals and control one's own body are basic to both the common sense and legal meaning of freedom. A basic premise of a free society is the right to oppose any sort of orthodoxy and act on this opposition. These ideals of freedom have long extended to beliefs about health and healing. Benjamin Rush, one of the signers of the Declaration of Independence, wrote, "The Constitution of the Republic should make special provision for Medical Freedom as well as Religious Freedom . . . to restrict the art of healing to one class of men and deny equal privileges to others will constitute the Bastille of medical science. All such laws are un-American and despotic. They are fragments of monarchy and have no place in a Republic."

Today it is commonplace to speak of the "right" to reject medical treatment or the "right" to die. The struggles of alternative medicine against the dominance of biomedicine fall squarely within this tradition. Practitioners feel they have the right to say what they believe is true and to act on those beliefs with other consenting adults. Those who use alternative therapies feel they have the right to control their bodies and to associate with whom they please. Most efforts to restrict the behavior of practitioners or users of alternative medicine can be viewed as a restriction of freedom and are used to create unity among a widely diverse group of providers, users, and potential users.

The importance of freedom as an overarching value for alternative medicine goes far beyond its connotation as a political right. It is the possibility of freedom that provides the basic justification for personal responsibility. It is our freedom which allows and demands that we be responsible for ourselves. Notions of "taking responsibility" for one's health in terms of behavior (stop smoking and start exercising) or consciousness (change your self-destructive thoughts and strengthen your immune system) are premised upon an assumption of freedom that is in tune with the most fundamental American values.

Advocates and practitioners of alternative medicine consistently promote freedom as a basic value in their work. Leaders like Weil, Burton Goldberg, and many others have often stressed that since different treatments work for different people suffering from the identical problem, everyone must have the freedom to chose their own treatment. If alternative medicine is to reach its potential, people must have free choice. One umbrella group, The National Health Federation (NHF) founded in 1955, states that its goal is "to protect our freedom to: eat fresh, clean food without pesticides, hormones, antibiotics, poisons, or irradiation; supplement our diets with vitamins, minerals, herbs, amino acids and enzymes; breathe clean air; use water free of toxic chemicals; choose a natural healer or allopathic doctor as we see fit. . . ." NHF's journal, *Health Freedom News,* offers information on a wide array of alternative therapies, almost always emphasizing one's first amendment right to use them and protesting the actions of various professional associations and the government to thwart them. Likewise, in their introduction to the compendium *Alternative Healing: The Complete A–Z Guide to More Than 150 Alternative Therapies,* the authors emphasize that a prerequisite to success "is that there should be freedom of choice in health care today and that an individual should know about these choices." In 1996, *Natural Health* magazine published a listing of "The 25 Best Books: Books that have changed our thinking about health and our world." For about half the books chosen, the editor's reason for selection was based upon the book's emphasis on expanding personal freedom. For example, they wrote: "For millions of people in their forties and fifties, *The Well Body Book* [a popular book by Mike Samuels and Hal Bennett, first published in 1973] marked a turning point in their lives. It told them 'you can be your own doctor.' Back then that was news to a lot of people." Asserting the importance of freedom is a central means of unifying the varied world of alternative medicine. Practitioners from very different backgrounds, who may have little knowledge or regard for each other's training or skills, can join together in asserting the right of clients to freely choose between them. Beyond its cultural resonance and grounding in traditional American values, the theme of free choice is a major element in establishing a common identity within the community of alternative medicine.

Over 150 years ago Max Weber described nineteenth century European capitalism as having an affinity with an ascetic eating style, based upon the belief that the overconsumption of food led to an inability to take on the responsibility of work. Similarly, physical exercise was thought to bring about piety, civility, leadership, and a reduced sexual drive. In America, these and similar ideas about economic success, personal responsibility, vigilance, and self control were echoed by Benjamin Franklin (in *Poor Richard's Almanac* and other writings), as well as by other health crusaders like Sylvester Graham, William Alcott, Ellen White, and the Kellogg brothers. Like the transcendentalists, such as Henry David Thoreau and Ralph Waldo Emerson, all these people saw prescriptions for exercise and diet as flowing directly from god. In the late 1800s a popular form of the gospel known as "muscular Christianity" swept the nation. It held that the form of the body could be perfected through exercise, leading to an improved quality of life and greater intelligence, as well as a better afterlife. As regular exercise made people more orderly, clear thinking, and exact, most of these leaders claimed financial success was also more likely. In the United States, freedom to control one's body has often been allied with the central focus of economic liberty.

Many of the organizations associated with alternative medicine have shown a marked affinity for the styles and values of entrepreneurial, small-scale capitalism very much like that expressed earlier in the nation's history. Today it is not difficult to find this convergence of values expressed in various alternative medical symposia, workshops, and writings. The 1997 Omega Institute catalogue offered programs such as "Creating the Work You Love: The Anti-Career Workshop." This workshop had the following description: "We receive powerful tools for turning our passions into viable projects, products and services . . . using a meditative format of exercises based on chakra systems . . . [to] confront our issues about abundance vs. scarcity, sharing vs. struggle. This technique, intended to align our inner world with outer manifestations, gives us the opportunity to create strategies for career development that are centered in the body, rather than trying to fit the body into a work situation. We uncover latent talents and priorities, devise strategies for self-employment, and develop a heart-centered prosperity."

The offerings at The Whole Life Expo (Pasadena, California, 1996) are considerably bolder in setting out this theme. The Expo's program guide offered a session entitled "Using PowerVision to Create Money Quickly" that it described as teaching participants "breakthrough PowerVision techniques for creating money quickly through expansive, spiritual energy! This instruction is from [the] . . . new motivating and inspiring book: *The Emergency Handbook for Getting Money Fast!*" The Expo also had talks on "How to Make a Million in Your Own Business in 5 Years or Less" and "Speed Wealth." The latter was described as "a step by step blueprint that allows current or aspiring entrepreneurs to make a million dollars or more in only 3–5 years. Most importantly, it shows them how to accomplish this objective while maintaining joy and balance in their lives. . . ." Deepak Chopra illustrates this connection of economics to alternative medicine quite vividly when he writes: ". . . when your actions are motivated by love . . . the surplus energy you gather and enjoy can be channeled to create anything you want, including unlimited wealth." The similarity between these descriptions' emphasis on economic freedom and the promises set out by many earlier American health movements is striking.

Describing "alternative medicine" as a cohesive entity in the United States of the late 1990s is still problematic, but increasingly less so than ever before. There has clearly been a rise in the use and acceptance of the term by the media, the government, the general public, conventional practitioners, and a wide array of nonconventional practitioners. Today "alternative medicine" reflects an existing reality well beyond that of the 1970s, when descriptions and commentary using the term were only beginning to appear.

The institutional and organizational base of alternative medicine that does exist is highly diverse and far from fully formed. The melange of publications, organizations, professional associations, and self promotions represent an emerging reality of alternative medicine, one that is highly fluid but nonetheless real. Professional associations and lobbying groups do exist, and they have already had some impact upon public policy and public perceptions. In part because of its rapid growth and eclectic character, the empirical world of alternative medicine does not exist as a fully mobilized or rational set of collective enterprises and actors, set to accomplish any clearly defined political goal. It is more of a "new social movement" where "actors self consciously practice in the present the future social changes they seek." The goals of the alternative medicine movement are as much about personal change as institutional change. There is a collective identity of those affiliated with alternative medicine, but it is a partial identity, coexisting and often in tension with other salient identities.

The institutions and organizations within alternative medicine are attempting to reduce the isolation between participants, raise a common consciousness, and develop both politically and organizationally. The extent of the movement's ability to mobilize itself over the past few years, as compared to the prior decade, is impressive.

6 The Politics of Alternative Medicine

Personal and Practical

Personal Politics

Although being healthy or sick is an intimate, highly personal experience, these states have a political dimension as well. The political overtones of alternative medicine have the potential to empower some people, while leaving others feeling powerless by linking guilt and self-blame to being ill.

Taking Responsibility

The political implications of alternative medicine's heavy emphasis on individual responsibility for health and healing have received intense scrutiny. Debate about the extent to which individual choice and personal responsibility are important in the cause and cure of illness dates back to Greek and Roman times. Alternative medicine's current prominence has renewed and deeply emphasized these questions. Almost every alternative school of healing and most well-known alternative healers stress the central role of questions like: "What sort of opportunity does this illness present for me to learn about myself?" and "What is it about my life choices, psychology, or wishes that has brought me to this point?" As one oft-cited phrase goes, "You are the Chairperson of your own well-being."

Despite the consistency of this theme within alternative medicine, there is a good deal of variation regarding precisely *what* one can or should be responsible for, or how people can

142

take more responsibility for their health. Alternative healers debate how much intentionality can be attributed to choice. Some acknowledge that people have a measure of control over behaviors such as using sunscreen or a seat belt. This represents a "mild" view that stresses the choices that people have but gives little blame or condemnation to those who are ill. On the other end of the spectrum are those who believe that people "chose to be born" and are responsible for everything that subsequently happens to them. According to the latter view, everyone "chooses" if they want to be healthy or ill and, likewise, they "choose" the specific illness and symptoms from which they suffer. People are considered to be wholly free and to have constant choices with certain consequences. If the consequences are not seen as emerging from free choice, their meaning cannot be comprehended and cure is beyond reach.

Carl Simonton is a very popular cancer doctor whose book *Choosing Cancer* typifies a moderate view. He writes, "All of us participate in becoming sick through a combination of mental, physical, and emotional factors. You may have neglected reasonable diet, exercise or rest. You may have been very tense or anxious for a long period of time without doing enough to relax. You may have maintained unreasonable workloads or gotten so caught up in meeting everyone else's needs that you ignored your own. You may have maintained attitudes and beliefs that prevented you from having satisfying emotional experiences. In sum, you may have failed to recognize your physical and emotional limits. To the extent that you ignored these legitimate needs, you participated in your own illness." Choosing to use the phrase "participate in," Simonton assigns people only partial responsibility for their health. Their own actions or psychological states contribute to disease but are not the sole cause of it.

A more extreme view speaks of "choosing" to be sick and intentionally damaging our bodies in order to achieve certain goals we can reach no other way. Proponents of this view blame those who don't "really want" to get well. As extreme as this perspective may sound, it is not difficult to find advocates who voice it. As Louise Hay, one best-selling author, put it:

> We are each 100% responsible for all our experiences. Every thought we think is creating our future. The point of power is always in the present moment. Everyone suffers from self-hatred and guilt. The bottom line for everyone is 'I'm not good enough.' It's only a thought, and a thought can be changed. Resentment, criticism, and guilt are the most damaging patterns. Releasing resentment will dissolve even cancer. When we really love ourselves, everything in our life works. We must release the past and forgive everyone. We must be willing to love ourselves. Self-approval and self-acceptance in the now are the key to positive changes. We create every so-called 'illness' in our body.

Hay's very successful books and workshops are devoted to expanding on each of these points, beginning with everyone's "choice" of their own parents. In a similar vein, Gerald Jampolsky says, "Slowly but surely, I am finding that nothing can hurt me except my own thoughts, my own mind," while C. Norman Shealy and Caroline Myss opine in *The Creation of Health* that "nothing, absolutely nothing, about our lives occurs outside of our personal power of choice." These ideas are typical of those holding an extreme view of choice and responsibility.

The extreme exponents of individual responsibility believe that other people or groups are constantly trying to thwart individuals from assuming control over their lives. To be healthy is to take (or take back) this power—to cast off the powerlessness that takes the form of illness. Thomas Szasz, a psychiatrist, has advocated this point of view with regard to the nature of illness and clearly drawn its political implications:

> First, there are those who want to take power away from the oppressor and give it to the oppressed, as a class. . . . Revealingly, they dream of the "dictatorship" of the proletariat or some other group.

Second, there are those who want to take power away from the oppressor and give it to themselves as the protectors of the oppressed—as exemplified by Robespierre in politics; Rush in medicine; and their liberal, radical, and medical followers. Revealingly, they dream of the incorruptibly honest or incontrovertibly sane ruler leading his happy or healthy flock.

And third, there are those who want to take power away from the oppressor and give it to the oppressed as individuals, for each to do with as he pleases, but hopefully for his own self-control—as exemplified by Mill, von Miss, the free market economists, and their libertarian followers. Revealingly, they dream of people so self-governing that their need and tolerance of rulers is minimal or nil.

While countless men say they love liberty, clearly only those who, by virtue of their actions, fall into the third category, mean it. The others merely want to replace a hated oppressor by a loved one, having usually themselves in mind for the job.

Szasz's view of individual responsibility is likely to lead to a political stance that minimizes the importance of social conditions in causing or exacerbating ill health. Issues such as poverty, racism, sexism, cultural patterns, environmental toxins, or lack of access to information and services are thought to be brought on and solvable by the independent action of individuals. As a practical matter, this view condemns government support for those who are sick, or at high risk, along with any sort of effort to reduce income inequality, discrimination, or poverty or enhance the well-being of children. The attitude is, "Why should I pay for someone else's bad choices?" But the political implications of these views go far beyond support of cost-cutting measures and cutbacks in aid to the poor. At least theoretically, these views have the potential to justify almost any sort of tyranny, repression, abuse, and even genocide. If *everyone* is responsible for *everything* that happens to them, children who are abused by their parents, or infants who die in an airplane crash, or victims of a repressive dictator all brought on their fate. Therefore, they must take responsibility for whatever has occurred. While few advocates of this extreme version of personal responsibility for health deal explicitly with health policy decision-making, their views have a marked affinity with the sorts of political forces that do.

There are even some who view the very use of scientific criteria to judge alternative medicine as an illegitimate form of political oppression. A scientific worldview values objectivity, quantification, universalism, intellectual abstraction, skepticism, and secularism. The scientist seeks absolutes that hold in a non-self-reflective way for everyone. On the other hand, the anti-science worldview proposes that the individual creates and is responsible for his or her universe. This view values subjectivity, qualitative data, egocentric views, uniqueness, accessibility to all, faith, and a disinterest in tests of falsifiability. Political groups that favor the latter set of values often advocate those alternative perspectives on health and illness that promote an extreme view of personal responsibility.

The affinity between far-right politics and alternative medicine goes well beyond the simple assumption that personal responsibility in social and economic life is conceptually similar to personal responsibility for health and illness. For example, a large "underground" of people and organizations, such as the Cancer Control Society, has long promoted "Laetrile" as an anti-cancer drug. Over the past three decades the group has staunchly advocated for a range of nutritional treatments along with various electromagnetic and other therapies for many serious chronic illnesses besides cancer, such as Lyme Disease, AIDS, and arthritis. The group is intimately tied to a number of clinics in Tijuana, Mexico, through promotions, travel arrangements, and the (sometimes illegal) importation of banned therapeutic agents for treatment. The leaders and many of the active members also support a heavily right-wing political agenda that centers on antipathy toward the federal government and its hostility to alternative cancer therapies. In 1996, the program of the 24th Annual Convention of the

Cancer Control Society included lectures on a wide variety of controversial alternative treatments (Hoxsey, Essiac, magnetism, shark cartilage, Laetrile) and on the political controversies surrounding alternative cancer care ("World Without Cancer— The Laetrile Story," "The FDA vs. Dr. Burzynski—Trial Update," "Alternative Medicine Lobbying 1997"). The Cancer Control Society's political stance specifically embodies Szasz's ideas about fighting those who would impose their "benign rationality" via state-sanctioned expertise to restrict the individual's right to take responsibility for his or her own health.

The agenda of the John Birch Society illustrates another overlap between a right-wing political agenda and support of alternative medicine. The motto of the John Birch Society "Less Government, More Responsibility, and—With God's Help—A Better World!" resonates with the emphasis on responsibility and spirituality that are so central to alternative medicine's worldview. Moreover, there is congruence between the John Birch Society's desire for less government and alternative medicine's interest in limiting government regulation of alternative health care products. This common interest is evident in the descriptions of the two health books available through the "health index" at the John Birch Society website. The website recommends one book, entitled *Alive and Well: One Doctor's Experience with Nutrition in the Treatment of Cancer Patients,* because it contains "many interesting and outrageous examples of the efforts of government and other health authorities to prevent [the doctor] from fulfilling the desire of patients to select the kind of treatment they desire." The focus is clearly political, and the story is one of government interference in the lives of individuals. However, in addition to the antiregulatory agenda of the book, the reviewer notes that it is "the story of an astonishing 20 year record of treating cancer patients with strict nutrition therapy" and includes an anti-cancer diet regimen. Thus, it is also the story of the value of alternative medicine in treating a life-threatening disease and familiarizes readers with the worldview of alternative medicine. The focus of the second book recommended by the John Birch Society is also bifurcated, on the one hand critiquing the federal government—in particular, the federal research agenda—and then also offering an alternative medical modality as the answer to a serious illness. The website reads, "This updated book re-examines the 'miracle' medicine Laetrile—a pure and concentrated form of Vitamin B17. When deficiency diseases, such as cancer, are treated with Laetrile, complete remission is possible. So why aren't these findings heralded on front page headlines? G. E. Griffin tells you why by exposing the politics of cancer research and the drug industry." Again, a link is made between government interference in individual freedom of choice and the practice of alternative medicine.

It is not difficult to find organizations and publications that combine alternative medicine advocacy with extreme, right-wing politics. The National Health Federation describes its mission as "to protect our freedom to: eat fresh, clean food without pesticides, hormones, antibiotics, poisons, or irradiation; supplement our diet with vitamins, minerals, herbs, amino acids and enzymes; breathe clean air; use water free of toxic chemicals; choose a natural healer or an allopathic doctor as we see fit; and to raise our children without dangerous drugs or vaccines, as we choose . . . to become self sufficient as possible in [our members'] quest for their personal best." The group's magazine, *Health Freedom News,* with a claimed readership of over 70,000, offers an amalgam of articles endorsing standard health promotion strategies ("have your blood pressure and cholesterol checked," "a working smoke detector is a must"), fairly sophisticated critiques of conventional medicine ("Do mammograms save women's lives?"), and advocacy of many alternative therapies ("Hemp Seed: the most nutritionally complete food source in the world"), along with harsh right-wing editorials ("THE ELECTION RECESS HAS ENDED. THE NATION IS ONCE AGAIN IN PERIL. . . . WHY DO WE HAVE A DEPARTMENT OF HEALTH, EDUCATION AND WELFARE??? LET'S ABOLISH THIS AGENCY").

Perceptions, a magazine published by the Betah Foundation to "expand opinion . . . in the areas of government, health, and metaphysics" goes even further. The March/April 1996 issue opens with an editorial supporting the idea that "the Federal Reserve is wholly owned by international bankers and . . . not one nickel of our personal income taxes pays for government services." Many of the articles take the stance that the federal government is not legitimate and that active resistance to it by withholding taxes or noncooperation with government agencies is the only way freedom can be maintained. Another article describes the "immense conspiracy" that has promoted the idea that the human race is exceptional in order to deny the overwhelming evidence of contact with humanoids from other planets. Feature articles on health take the position that "mad cow disease" is caused by canola oil and that mercury in dental fillings is partly responsible for both Alzheimer's disease and cardiovascular disease. In each case, the magazine offers a conspiracy theory holding the government, especially the FDA and the medical profession, responsible for the problem. The piece on canola oil concludes, "It should come as no surprise that anyone wanting to enjoy peak health and longevity *must* take personal control of and responsibility for his or her health and life. There is *no* other way! 'Health care industry' is an oxymoron. . . . Learn to protect *your* health and economic interests by learning how to take care of yourself. Then act on that knowledge." Within the world of those who subscribe to this publication, these positions are moderate. The advertisements are dominated by both purveyors of alternative therapies and support services for the extreme right wing ("the Patriot Matchmaker . . . the ultimate in preparedness, [will] help you find a patriot/survivalist minded partner to survive the uncertainties of the 1990's and the year 2000 plus. We all know the difficulties of relating to the uninformed. . . .").

In addition to sharing an emphasis on personal responsibility for health, both political conservatism and alternative medicine hope to reintroduce religion and spirituality into daily life and public discourse. Statements about spirituality and faith permeate the literature of the new conservatives. President Ronald Reagan, in his famous "Evil Empire" address to the National Association of Evangelicals in 1981, stated his belief that "the real crisis . . . we are facing today is a spiritual one. . . . At root, it is a test of moral will and faith." A similar set of ideas about faith and partnership with god are also central to the theories of many alternative healers. As Jampolsky stated, "To me, healing is letting God write the script of my life. It is choosing to let God's will and my will be one." There is little doubt that an affinity exists between alternative medicine's stance regarding personal responsibility for health and healing and the views of those who advocate conservative political values.

Despite the empirical affinity of conservative politics with notions about personal responsibility for health, these same ideas are also compatible with left-wing political perspectives. Many observers have noted that members of groups involved with Eastern religions and health practices like yoga and meditation frequently hold "liberal" political views that stress moral relativism and an openness to a multiplicity of cultural values. Those adopting these views and practices often come from elite, sophisticated, urban backgrounds where liberal politics are more common.

As on the right, one can find extreme versions of the amalgamation of individual responsibility and left-wing views. Many far-left and revolutionary political groups have held an antipositivist view of social change along with their empirically based critiques on the distribution of rewards in society. From this perspective, it is people's ability to imagine different social arrangements that initially motivates and creates social change. Thus, on a conceptual basis, taking responsibility for personal empowerment can result in political empowerment. Personal responsibility can lead to both personal and social revolution. The work of Paolo Freire, the radical Brazilian educational "missionary" among the poor, exemplifies this orientation toward personal responsibility as the harbinger of revolutionary change. Freire's approach is based on the idea that oppressed people have "introjected" a "slave consciousness" into the deeper recesses of their being. Liberation depends on "extrojecting" it. In *Pedagogy of the Oppressed* Freire writes, "I was convinced that the Brazilian people could learn social and political responsibility only by *experiencing* that responsibility. . . . They could be helped to learn democracy through the exercise of democracy; for that knowledge, above all others, can only be assimilated experientially. . . . We needed . . . an education which would lead men to take a new stance towards their problems—that of intimacy with those problems [and] principles." Based upon these views, Freire and his followers are highly supportive of most forms of indigenous health practice as a means by which oppressed groups can control more of what affects them. For Freire, professionally constructed explanations for problems and professionally controlled therapies only reinforce the oppressed community's sense of powerlessness.

The political implications of individual responsibility for health and illness in alternative medicine are highly plastic. There is potential for resonance between an emphasis on personal responsibility for health and most any political perspective. Extremists, both those on the right and left, have been drawn to it and utilize it for their own ends. Currently, those on the political right are more likely to invoke the values of alternative medicine in their belief that collective action, especially on the part of the government, cannot resolve social problems. It is true that an emphasis on personal responsibility is a common feature of just about every alternative mode of health care. But that consistency shouldn't obscure the fact that this focus on personal responsibility has been thoroughly "Americanized." It is joined to our existing cultural norms of individualism ("take charge"), sexism ("its all in your head, so either just cut it out, or take some Valium to get rid of it"), and general medical judgmentalism. In its original Eastern context, the emphasis on individual responsibility is buffered by the belief that what goes on within the physical and mental ecology of the individual is a direct reflection of the broader social and physical environment outside the individual. Thus while a person must be responsible for his or her illness in the sense of accepting its reality and dealing with it, that does not imply that he or she caused it. In this sense, a belief in personal responsibility can be utilized as a "humane" justification for reducing or increasing expectations about what people can and cannot do.

Empirical studies have generally concluded that the potential for alternative medicine's focus on individual responsibility to foster or exacerbate strong political views is seldom realized in clinical practice. While those who hold specific political views to begin with may seek healers or settings that emphasize this synergism, most alternative practitioners, clinics, and groups are apolitical. Regardless of an ideology that may allow "blaming the victim" for not trying hard enough, or even "not wanting" to get well if a cure is not achieved, there is little or no evidence that alternative clinicians are more punitive than conventional doctors. In her study of alternative physicians, nurses, and psychologists June Lowenberg found that "these holistic health practitioners *do* absolve" and that the providers were very aware of the danger of assigning blame for illness or the lack of a cure. Instead, practitioners used a variety of interpretations, such as redefining intent ("you couldn't control what you were doing if you didn't know it was gonna lead you to this") to minimize the burden on the patient. The mission statement of the Research Center for Alternative Medicine typifies this approach by emphasizing personal responsibility for health as a by-product of "understanding mind-body integration." The implication clearly is that without such understanding, there can be no real responsibility for illness.

Community Empowerment and Coalitions

Despite the attention it receives, personal responsibility for health and illness is not the only aspect of alternative medicine's core beliefs that has political implications. Many interest groups that seek to build "identity" or "community" as a means of gaining political power in society have taken to alternative medicine's idea of personal responsibility for health and emphasis on wholeness or unity as an organizing principle. There has been an association between American feminism and various forms of alternative healing since the early nineteenth century. A belief in spiritual healing and the power of the mind to influence the body offered a sense of personal empowerment to women who sought to break free of the legal power that men held over them. Today the women's health movement is replete with themes similar to those found in best-selling alternative medicine books. The preface of the popular and influential book *The New Our Bodies, Ourselves* begins by embracing the idea of personal responsibility for health. The authors describe the book's goal as "to reach as many women as possible with the tools that will enable them to take greater charge of their own health care and their lives, deal with the existing medical system and fight whenever possible for improvements and changes." The remainder of the book, which has now sold millions of copies, presents the necessity of synthesizing mind, body, and spirit (termed "feminism") when dealing with any of the full range of health issues and problems that affect women. The overall goal is the development of a communitarian "feminist" identity and collective action. But the means to attain these ends utilize the same core values of holism and the integration of body mind and spirit that permeate alternative medicine. Throughout the book, the authors voice skepticism about the medical profession, especially its reliance upon high technology for diagnosis and treatment. "Natural" or low technology—such as using unpasteurized yogurt douches to prevent vaginal infections—is encouraged, and there is a very strong emphasis on health promotion through diet and exercise as a means of preventing illness and restoring health.

The gay liberation movement has used the idea of individual responsibility to build group cohesion in a manner similar to the women's movement. The impact of the AIDS epidemic on the gay community has also politicized many gays and lesbians regarding health issues: The gay and lesbian community discovered that the system of health care delivery was filled with racism, homophobia, sexism, and classism. In response, they created scores of organizations to provide compassionate health care alternatives for people with HIV. The AIDS Coalition To Unleash Power (ACT-UP) is a dramatic and frequently cited example of gays taking responsibility on themselves to mobilize in response to the popular perception that the government and traditional health care institutions were moving too slowly in recognizing and combating the AIDS epidemic. This group strengthened the unity of the gay liberation movement as a whole. These examples of the gay and women's health movements suggest an affinity between values of alternative medicine and the strategies used by many non-mainstream groups to enhance their cohesiveness and build power and unity among their members.

Feminist and gay groups that have attained increasing presence and recognition in the larger society tend to be quite comfortable with much of the underlying premises of alternative medicine. Whatever their politics, women who have been in consciousness-raising groups or the chronically ill who have been in support groups will probably find that much of the alternative medical perspective is not "alien" or "foreign." The core values of alternative medicine increasingly are not seen as the sole property of alternative medicine. They belong to a set of social movements and "identity groups," many of which have liberal or progressive political views.

A similar overlap can be seen between alternative medicine's core values and orientation toward health found among certain American ethnic groups. Beliefs about the unity of mind, body, and spirit—as well as vitalism—and the presence of energy forces throughout life are central to the beliefs of numerous groups from Asia and Latin America. Many people from these backgrounds currently practice culturally based, nonmainstream medicine. These groups represent a rapidly increasing proportion of immigrants in the United States and are highly concentrated in certain geographic regions, providing a receptive base for alternative therapies. The alternative medical community is well aware of this potential. Many alternative practitioners are usually well acquainted with the foreign roots and history of the techniques they employ, along with the mutual benefit to be derived from fostering a broad legal and cultural acceptance of alternative approaches.

Thus, the underlying values of alternative medicine are congruous with those found in a wide array of political perspectives and groups. The oft-stated affinity of alternative medicine's emphasis on personal responsibility with conservative groups is real. But personal responsibility is also a point of convergence with many progressive groups that are involved with identity politics: women, gays and lesbians, ethnic minorities, the disabled, and others. These same groups are also quite comfortable with many other central aspects of alternative medicine.

Counter-Culture Politics

Since the late 1960s, the term "counter-culture" has been used to describe those who challenge certain aspects of mass industrial society. The term is vague, referring to discrete groups of individuals who choose a specific lifestyle, as well as to an amorphous set of values and styles manifest in popular culture, especially in music, dress, and the use of psychoactive drugs. Some of the most consistent values espoused by those who identify as "counter-cultural" are an antipathy toward high technology and the distrust of conventional bureaucratic institutions, experts, and objectivity. In this regard, the concerns of the counter-culture overlap those of alternative medicine, with its emphasis on the primacy of low tech and "natural" solutions, personal responsibility, and altered states of consciousness. The use of invasive techniques—especially those with iatrogenic consequences such as radiation, surgery, and chemotherapy—is an anathema to both counter-cultural and alternative perspectives.

The use of "mind expanding" or psychoactive drugs is an important area of overlap between alternative medicine and the counter-culture. During the early 1960s, Timothy Leary, Richard Alpert, and other psychologists, many at Harvard University, popularized the use of LSD and other psychedelic drugs and described the experience in terms of Buddhist and Taoist concepts. The widespread use of these drugs, along with marijuana, became both a symbolic and an actual representation of a "counter-culture" that encompassed underground newspapers, food co-ops, free schools, and numerous free clinics and women's health centers. All these locations provided settings and opportunities for people to become familiar with many types of alternative medicine, including acupuncture, herbal remedies, massage, shamanism, and meditative techniques. By 1970, Alpert had changed his name to Baba Ram Dass and was teaching yoga, meditation, and nutrition along with the best ways to get high on drugs. Ram Dass remains involved with the alternative health movement, frequently teaching at the workshops of the Omega Institute and disseminating his teachings on spirituality and health through his "Hanuman Foundation" mail order library. Following Ram Dass's stroke in 1997, many well-known advocates and teachers of mind-body medicine and alternative healing volunteered to staff a retreat at the Omega Institute, with the net proceeds going to a fund for his care and recovery. Creating altered states of consciousness, whether through drugs or by other means such as meditation or hypnosis, was central to both the counter-culture's view of what was desirable and pleasurable, and to the alternative medical view of what people needed to assume control over their own health and future.

By the late 1970s, many aspects of the counter-culture had receded or been trivialized by commercialism and other forces. But the "free clinics" continued to expand, often focusing their efforts on poor and marginalized groups such as the homeless along with their traditional counter-cultural clientele. This environment continued to provide a setting where a de facto integration of alternative and conventional medical approaches could occur. Although some of these clinics used alternative techniques for a limited range of problems, often related to drug abuse treatment, other centers developed as full "holistic" or alternative medical clinics. The longstanding and ongoing connection between the worldviews of the counter-culture and alternative medicine had influenced both parties. Those who came from the free clinics and the counter-culture were generally liberal and progressive in their political views. They believed alternative medical approaches would foster their goals and viewed their emphasis on altered states of consciousness as a positive attribute, if only for its potentially pleasurable aspects. More importantly, groups that felt themselves to be disenfranchised or powerless saw that they could use alternative beliefs and techniques to gain control over their bodies and health. At the same time, those who came from the world of alternative medicine saw those with very liberal politics strongly supporting and using their ideas and practices.

One recent manifestation of this linkage is the movement to legalize marijuana to relieve symptoms of AIDS, cancer, glaucoma, and other conditions. A coalition of counter-cultural and alternative medical groups played leading roles in the successful effort to get Proposition 215, which legalized such use under very loose controls, on the 1996 ballot and approved by California voters. Proposition 215 supporters presented the campaign as a criticism of mainstream medicine's refusal to use a natural substance that was clinically effective. Support for the legal use of marijuana for medical purposes cuts across political lines. A 1997 CBS News poll found that 57 percent of Republicans as well as 64 percent of Democrats and 66 percent of independents supported the idea. But the subtext and the actual operation of the initiative has been to reinforce the broader goal of the legalization of marijuana for recreational use. Andrew Weil strongly supports marijuana's medical value. But he also considers conventional medicine's views about marijuana as "not rational" and advises visitors to his website to read a number of books that call for marijuana's "full legalization under the same rules that are applied to alcohol." Given Weil's oft-expressed position that humans have an innate desire, as basic as the need for food, to experience altered states of consciousness, his views about marijuana are no surprise. His goal is to teach people how to improve their minds by moving from "straight" to "stoned" thinking. In much of his work Weil is quite explicit about the attraction all sorts of alternative medicine movements have had to those who hold an antiauthoritarian stance.

Currently, a portion of the alternative medical community strongly supports building upon the sorts of relationships that existed with the free clinics to create a "green" medicine, after the name of the progressive European political movement. Dana Ullman, a well-known advocate of homeopathy, and other advocates of this position emphasize alternative medicine's view that symptoms do not necessarily mean that something is wrong with the individual as much as they indicate a response of the organism to stress or to some other factor in the broader environment. This ecological view of health and illness is one key potential link of the worldview of progressive politics and alternative medicine. Ullman makes the point that recognizing the way in which economic forces can permeate the individual's health fits quite nicely with the belief that various forms of energy transverse the body via a set of invisible pathways. While this sort of amalgamation of perspectives has been infrequent, it is tenable.

Practical Politics

Regardless of the political implications that its core beliefs may hold for the broader society, alternative medicine has a set of more mundane political goals. These matters involve the certification of alternative practitioners; official government recognition, if not approval of various alternative therapies; the use of government funds for the delivery of alternative medicine; and the training of alternative practitioners. How these issues are eventually resolved will in large measure determine whether, and in what form, alternative medicine is integrated into the mainstream of American medicine. For example, it is this set of essentially political decisions that will determine if Medicare and private insurance plans will reimburse their members for alternative medicine and precisely *which* providers can be reimbursed for *what*. Given the stakes, it is not surprising that these questions are of major concern to those who practice and use alternative therapies, as well as those who are opposed to their acceptance. Within the world of alternative medicine there is a common understanding that these goals can only come about through a set of political actions. Those furthest from the mainstream seek to maximize "medical freedom of choice," disestablish the Food and Drug Administration ("medical establishment cops"), and halt the "concerted effort on the part of government regulatory agencies to punish and harass" alternative practitioners along with "state medical boards who censure and revoke the licenses of conscientious physicians who practice alternative medicine." Yet even proponents of such "extreme" views understand that these matters can only be accomplished through practical politics.

Certification and Credentialing

The question of *who* has the legal authority to do *what* (along with the matter of who cannot do what) is one of the most complicated and vexing of all the political issues surrounding alternative medicine. A coherent public policy requires that both the "who" and the "what" be defined. Those who seek a broad certification or credential for something on the order of an "alternative" or "holistic" physician/healer must first operationalize these terms. Given the difficulty in reaching a consensus on the meaning of these terms, this is likely to be a complex, if not fruitless, undertaking. Defining more narrowly drawn types of alternative providers such as massage therapists or acupuncturists is much easier, assuming a consensus exists on a common base of knowledge, skills, and training. Yet for most types of alternative therapy the development of such a consensus has barely begun. These definitional problems are exacerbated by the demands of many existing groups of health care professionals who want to subsume the practice of alternative therapies under the mandate of their own existing licensure. "Chaotic" would accurately describe the current situation with regard to certification and credentialing. The chaos is heightened by the sense that the situation may be rapidly changing as the public and policymakers have begun to see a need to rectify the situation. Decisions arrived at now may strongly influence the forms of alternative medical practice for some time to come.

Licensure, Power and Being a Professional

Power and autonomy are almost always underlying issues when licensure and certification are discussed, and this is surely the case with regard to alternative medicine. Will licensure grant the autonomy and self-regulation that is the sociological hall-mark of true "professions," or will it lock practitioners into the much more limited roles of "paraprofessionals," working under the control of some other authority? Not surprisingly, practitioners themselves typically seek to maximize their professional status and authority. Existing groups of professionals within mainstream medicine who already possess broad authority will tend to resist the demands of insurgent groups as will those, like insurance companies, who have to pay the higher fees that autonomous professionals are better able to command. The granting of professional autonomy through licensure is always a highly political process. The conflict over the granting of professional autonomy and prerogatives is especially intense at a time such as the present when the autonomy of most existing professional groups, particularly physicians, is becoming more restricted by the institutions of "managed care." Along with market forces, the ability of alternative practitioners to get the political powers to accept their core beliefs as legitimate will be crucial in the outcome of their struggle for recognition. Currently, they are at the earliest stage of this process.

The American Holistic Medical Association (AHMA) was formed in 1978, initially restricting its membership to physicians, osteopaths, and medical students. Later, responding to its inability to grow, it added associate memberships for all "state licensed holistically oriented practitioners, such as chiropractors, naturopaths, nurses, psychologists, dentists, etc." The organization's leaders have come to recognize that regardless of the AHMA's ability to offer support and education to its members, any future growth (membership has been fairly constant at about seven hundred) depends upon the ability to "establish the American Board of Holistic Medicine and become a certified medical specialty." The group has proposed a core curriculum of seven areas (nutritional medicine, physical activity, environmental medicine, behavioral medicine, social health, energy medicine, and spiritual atonement) for training and examination. Botanical medicine, bimolecular therapy, ethno medicine (TCM, Ayurveda, Native American), and manual medicine are listed as potential subspecialties. The board eventually wants to offer more limited certification for non-physicians. In essence, the AHMA's future is dependent upon its ability to forge an internal consensus on what it means to be a holistic physician, and to use that consensus as a means of gaining political recognition. The AHMA's hope is that recognition of the board it created would eventually allow it to certify those who practice within that definition.

The American Holistic Nursing Association (AHNA) has taken a very different approach, expanding its initially exclusive focus on nurses to include anyone interested "in holistically oriented health care practices" and eschewing the endorsement of any core knowledge base, certification process, or modality of healing. Its mission is to "Create opportunities for nurses to heal and empower ourselves and others through modeling and integrating holism in lives and practices." It has an active membership of about four thousand. Groups like the American Association for Holistic Health are even less specific about membership criteria (anyone can join) and present themselves essentially as clearinghouses for monitoring legislation and promoting a broad acceptance of holistic health care.

Each of these alternative medical organizations faces a common dilemma. They all share the overall goal of increasing the acceptance of alternative medicine. Official recognition via licensure and quasi-official recognition through board certification would greatly facilitate the recognition they seek, along with improvements in status and income. But the various groups involved have very different needs and desires. For already licensed professions, a broad certification as a "holistic physician," or dentist, or psychologist would be desirable. But groups like massage therapists or reflexologists need a much more limited mandate. Other groups, such as chiropractors or nurses, already have a license that grants a limited, though significant, degree of autonomy. Such groups tend to be split into those who find the current state of affairs acceptable and those who seek a much broader degree of autonomy and professional self-control.

The situation is further complicated by the fact that many alternative practitioners utilize more than one modality of care. For example, some chiropractors seeking to expand their services are now practicing homeopathy as well. Only a small number of these obtain any sort of homeopathic certification, and most see their basic training in chiropractic as inclusive enough to allow them to self-train in homeopathy, as well as in nutritional therapy and other techniques. As primary health care providers, the chiropractors expect to be treated the same as conventional physicians, who have wide leeway in choosing which modes of treatment to utilize. Under some proposals, a recognized certification for practicing homeopathy might disqualify chiropractors or physicians from using it. Each group of professionals will have very different opinions about what is in its best interest. Organizations whose goal is the advancement of homeopathy (as opposed to homeopaths) such as the National Center for Homeopathy may find it expedient to side with neither group of providers. This lack of *internal* cohesiveness regarding basic skills, training, and interrelationships with other health care providers is a major current impediment to the credentialing of alternative providers.

In this regard the situation facing alternative providers today is much like the one allopathic physicians faced at the turn of the century. As Paul Starr has described, medicine was able to secure autonomy from the government through licensure via a small group of physicians' consolidation of authority over decision-making and political alliances. It had nothing to do with the validity of biomedical theories or the utility of medical therapies. It was this consolidated leadership that allowed the vision of scientific medicine to triumph over an array of competing views and forge the political links necessary to enact the desired prerogatives into law. The creation of internal cohesion was carried out with both "the carrot and the stick." Almost all the existing physicians, regardless of training or skill, were granted credentials as long as those who were judged deficient agreed to give up any claims to control within the new profession.

If a group is to successfully attain even limited recognition and licensure for its work, it requires an internal consensus sufficient to engage in a unified lobbying campaign. Typically, the legislative agenda of these campaigns is to establish standards for entering the field, in the form of training and supervised field experience, and to create a licensing board that has the power to control entry into, and discipline over, the group. Consensus among the initial practitioners, many of whom do not have the formal training and supervised experience necessary to qualify, is achieved by "grandfathering" them in. Often, older practitioners become the gatekeepers into the profession and run the training programs through which new recruits enter the field. As the field grows, the requirements for entry can be made more rigorous, thus holding down the number of competitors and keeping economic rewards relatively high. Every group of health care providers in the history of the nation has followed this pattern. A consensus among providers allows for the imposition of restrictions and limitations on the scope of practice in exchange for autonomy and control, if not monopolization, over a limited set of activities or area of knowledge. The process is encapsulated by the comments of Ann Davis, a massage therapist from Memphis who led the Tennessee Massage Therapy Association and Tennessee chapter of the American Massage Therapy Association in their successful quest to license massage therapy in that state. After the law (which provides for a licensing board and five hundred hours of basic training) was passed, she said, "One of the most outstanding features of the Act is that we own the term 'massage' and the professional term 'massage therapist'—someone cannot even imply that they are using massage techniques without becoming licensed. It's a good, strong law."

While the creation of credentials for broadly conceived alternative healers is mired in definitional and jurisdictional conflicts, the official recognition of a wide array of specific alternative health providers is rapidly, if confusingly, proceeding. Many groups such as chiropractors, optometrists, psychologists, and midwives already have widely accepted credentials that license them to conduct a restricted range of procedures, sometimes while nominally supervised by a physician. This sort of licensure offers the possibility of a limited and tentative entry into the mainstream health care system, often with some right to be reimbursed by insurance companies. Typically, a group that accepts this limited sort of licensure formally gives up its claim to be primary general health care providers in exchange for this circumscribed acceptance. Although some groups (such as homeopaths) or factions of groups (such as those chiropractors who refuse to restrict their practice to spinal manipulation) may reject these limited victories, many groups of alternative providers eagerly pursue them.

Professional self-interest is not the only factor pushing toward the growth of limited licensure and certification of alternative providers. As the various alternative approaches become more widely known, even those who oppose them find themselves calling for standardization. When *Consumer Reports* published an extremely negative article on homeopathy, one of its major complaints was that "there are no uniform training standards for people learning homeopathy." The piece concluded that the absence of these standards for certification is of much greater concern to the public than the consumer advocacy magazine's finding of no theoretical or empirical basis for the homeopathy itself.

As homeopathy and many other alternative therapies rapidly increase their visibility and presence in society, forces urging certification and licensure are growing quickly. But the American political system, where licensure and certification are the responsibility of fifty states and a bewildering maze of regulatory jurisdictions, prevents the process from going forward in a consistent manner. More than eleven hundred different health-related occupations are now regulated, six hundred by full licensure, by the various states. But about half the states regulate fewer than sixty different occupations. In these states, over a thousand health-related job titles are completely unregulated. Chiropractors are the only alternative providers licensed in every state, with equal rights to reimbursement as physicians in forty-five states. Acupuncturists are licensed in twenty-eight states (with licensure pending in nine more and regulations governing acupuncture in most others), naturopaths in eleven states (two pending), and massage therapists in four (with twenty-four states considering some sort of regulation). Chiropractors, acupuncturists, and naturopaths are the only groups whose training is accredited by the U.S. Department of Education.

In 1994, the Fetzer Institute commissioned David Sale, an attorney, to write "An Overview of Legislative Developments Concerning Alternative Health Care in the United States," which reviewed provider practice legislation for twenty-seven different alternative therapies, the medical practice acts of seven states, and various pieces of federal legislation. Sale found that states differ widely in which therapies they recognize and whether they deal with them via licensure, registration, or certification. There is no consistency in this rapidly growing arena other than an intensification of legislative effort in most states. Sale did find that state legislation has allowed those groups that are already most well established (physicians, chiropractors, naturopaths, acupuncturists) to consolidate their existing power by adding on a wide range of alternative modalities, regardless of any indication of skill or training. He also found that many less well-known modes of treatment—such as bioenergetics, polarity therapy, reflexology, Rolfing, and Hellerwork—are beginning to appear in legislation. In many cases, securing the right to practice one form of treatment is associated with "cross-practice" rights, which he felt reflects the "fluidity" of the area. His most important conclusion was that the overall lack of consistency is fast creating a pressing need for some sort of federal intervention, at least at the consensus building level. Some sort of "model" legislation is needed, and this will require more governmental attention to the efficacy of alternative medicine.

Evaluating Alternative Approaches

Despite the growing desire of alternative practitioners to gain state-sanctioned credentials and licensure, most of the political pressure for dealing with alternative approaches has come from critics outside the field. The critics are primarily concerned with establishing the safety and effectiveness of particular treatments that have attracted popular attention. Typically, the pattern of consumer use and governmental interest in regulation develops as follows: Advocates make a claim about some treatment or preventive strategy (e.g., shark cartilage is effective in treating or preventing cancer). A growing number of individuals engage in the behavior and attest to its benefits. The mass media report on the phenomenon. They note the technique's popularity and the amount of money being spent on it but stress that there is really very little objective data to support any sort of conclusion as to its merit. Almost inevitably, the media calls for government-sponsored research on the topic and legislation or regulation to ensure product standardization and consumer safety.

A 1995 *Newsweek* article on herbal remedies—"Sex, Lies, and Garlic"—is typical of hundreds of similar pieces in the national news media. It largely dismisses claims for the benefits of melatonin, ginseng root, wheat grass, and dozens of other herbal remedies as anecdotal. At the same time, it summarizes this list of claims in tabular form, noting the contraindications for each ("ginkgo biloba . . . overdose can cause nausea or diarrhea") and listing the most popular name brands for each one. The article concludes that commercial products are "notoriously uneven." It notes, for example, that some studies have found a fourth of the products sold as ginseng to contain no ginseng at all, while other studies have found tenfold variations in ginseng potency. The language of the article decries that lack of standardization and suggests caution, while the visual presentation serves as a shoppers' guide.

Another example of how media criticism may promote government recognition of alternative approaches is a 1996 *New York Times* series of large, front-page articles entitled "Alternative Medicine: Beyond the Mainstream." Alternative medicine is described as "an unconventional approach to health embraced by its followers but criticized by many physicians and scientists." The first of the lengthy articles—"On Fringes of Health Care, Untested and Unregulated Therapies Thrive"—was quite hostile to the claims of any therapeutic value for alternative therapy, particularly for nutritional supplements. A large portion of the article is devoted to graphs showing the growth in annual sales of the four largest publicly traded companies that sell nutritional supplements (in 1991 approximately $620 million, in 1995 over $1 billion), and the simultaneous escalation in the stock prices of these firms. The article concluded that the reason for this growth was the dismantling of federal regulation for naturally occurring substances, commonly called food or dietary supplements. Now, as long as their advertising claims are not on the packages themselves, these products are immune from regulation. This deregulation came about largely through the efforts of Senator Orrin Hatch of Utah, a conservative who has long advocated for "freedom of choice" in health care and promoted the interests of the large natural foods industry in his home state.

The article closed with a call for more research on and regulation of food supplements. It ended with a quote from the oncologist who was then president of the American Cancer Society: "When you examine how much money is spent you should really demand that there is some evidence for what you are receiving." Regulation of alternative medicine is one form of governmental recognition of the field.

The advocates of regulation have used the faddish popularity of the herb ephedra to press their case. Sold under the name "herbal ecstasy," some of those who marketed it claimed it would produce euphoria, sexual simulation, and an overall legal "high." Although it had long been sold in health food stores and marketed as a weight loss aid and energy enhancer, some firms began to sell high dose versions over the Internet, in "head shops," and other places where teenagers congregate. News reports claimed that the herb was responsible for as many as fifteen overdose deaths among teens, although firm documentation of these numbers was difficult to find. The FDA was unable to respond effectively because, as a food product, the herb did not require any labeling about its safety or impact. An op-ed piece in the *New York Times* about the abuse of ephedra depicted it as an outgrowth of the lack of regulation for "natural foods and substances" like melatonin. The author of the article, a physician, queried, "How long will it be before Congress realizes the dangers of unregulated toxic products?" and concluded that Congress should "give the FDA back its authority to regulate all drugs and dietary supplements, 'natural' as well as synthetic." Since the active ingredient in the herb, ephedrine, has long been sold over the counter with FDA approval in dozens of asthma remedies, and as pseudoephedrine in hundreds of cold and sinus remedies, it is possible that the concern about ephedra might arise from a more basic desire to regulate other nutritional substances. In June of 1997, the FDA decided that ephedra did pose a "health risk" and issued compromise regulations that limited tablets to no more than 8 milligrams and required stronger warning labels on packages.

One of the best known examples of the efforts of those outside alternative medicine to seek regulatory control over the substances used by nonconventional therapists is the case of Dr. Stanislaw Burzynski. A Polish-born physician with a Ph.D. in biochemistry, Burzynski was well on his way to a career in academic medicine at the Baylor College of Medicine in Houston when, in 1973, he and another physician colleague reported very promising effects of peptides to inhibit the growth of cancer cells. The work proved highly controversial. It was based upon Burzynski's application of an established clinical insight that people with renal failure, who overproduce peptides, almost never get cancer. But the study also enraged his colleagues because it was carried out in the Department of Anesthesiology, as opposed to one of the departments that usually sponsored cancer-related research. As soon as Burzynski's funding from the National Cancer Institute ran out (his follow-up proposal was approved but did not score high enough to be funded), he was forced out of Baylor and continued his work with private funding. After an initial trial with twenty-one severely ill cancer patients proved quite successful, he began to charge fees from patients at his clinic for what he openly called an "experimental" treatment. This, and his ongoing efforts to seek out and accept seriously ill cancer patients to be treated by his methods (almost always after referral by their own doctors who had given up hope for them), led the FDA to file an array of charges against him. The cases dragged on for over fourteen years and led to a convoluted set of counter-claims by Burzynski and his supporters about the use of intimidation by federal agents, along with a great deal of attention from the mass media.

Despite the tirade of extremely critical comments directed toward his methods, theory, and findings, none of the charges brought against Burzynski by the government, the established medical profession, or the FDA ever specified any scientific deficiencies in his work. The government's entire case was premised on his violation of established medical "ethics" by charging for an experimental treatment and his unwillingness to share the formula for his treatment with other researchers. In all the attacks on him, no effort was ever made to scientifically refute any of his findings. Burzynski was never found guilty in any court of any charge. In May of 1997, he was acquitted of the last of seventy-five charges of mail fraud and interstate delivery of an unapproved drug. By exemplifying the fight against governmental regulation as a means of restricting nonconventional therapies for political reasons, his case became a major *cause célèbre* among advocates of many forms of alternative therapy.

The greatest long-term significance of the Burzynski case may be that it motivated almost all the parties, regardless of their initial stance, to seek political clarification of the rights of alternative practitioners. The courts repeatedly found that the controls exerted by regulatory agencies, and by the mainstream medical profession, had violated the rights of Burzynski and his patients. The Burzynski case also points out the importance of national legislation in this area. The majority of charges leveled against him had to do with interstate commerce: promoting and shipping the drugs he developed from one state to another. He was fully licensed in Texas, but this meant little in other states.

This situation is typical with regard to the regulation of other alternative healing techniques. The various states offer a patchwork of regulations that are sometimes contradictory in impact. For example, twenty states regulate acupuncture, but some define it in terms of needle insertion, others as an attempt to control energy flows in the body. Still others regulate it as part of the practice and licensure of "Oriental medicine." Similarly, twenty-two states regulate massage, each defining it to include different techniques. Some states include techniques such as polarity therapy, Trager bodywork, or reflexology as part of massage; others specifically exclude them. Given the lack of conceptual or pragmatic justification for the existing laws, the overall sense is one of chaos and confusion. Increasingly, the paramount need of all interested parties (clients and potential clients, insurers, practitioners, etc.) is to have at least minimal consistency in defining the range of alternative modalities and who can practice them. As conventional physicians, out of belief or client pressure, become more likely to refer clients for alternative therapy, they too find themselves requiring the clarity that legislation and accepted credentialing can offer.

The need to balance the demands of innovators for a piece of the action with the desire of existing groups to keep their power is much like that which has occurred with "organic" food. The vagueness of the term, combined with the growing popularity of the concept, resulted in intense confusion in the marketplace. In late 1997 when the federal government finally issued standards for food being called "organic," it was only after decades of pressure from those who produced such food. But just like acupuncturists or homeopaths who successfully lobby for legal recognition of their therapy only to find that the new law gives control over it to physicians, the new definition of "organic" was written in a way to favor existing giant agribusiness firms. Only a massive outpouring of criticism from the producers, sellers, and users of "real" organic food forced some revisions that again favored the smaller, long-time producers of organic food.

Federal Legislation

With regard to national legislation, the United States lags behind most western European nations as well as China and Japan. These countries have longstanding mechanisms for conducting research on herbs and other alternative techniques, as well as centralized bodies for accrediting training programs and certifying practitioners. In Germany, "Commission E" (an official government agency) regularly informs all physicians about research on herbal medicines. In Britain, Prince Charles's personal involvement in alternative medicine led to the formation of several quasi-governmental commissions with the express task of integrating alternative medicine into the National Health Service. The twenty-five nations that make up the European Commission have been conferring on standardizing these practices since 1992. Not only do American physicians, researchers, regulators, and health planners lag far behind their European counterparts in these matters, they are largely ignorant of how far behind they are.

In the United States, there is minimal national legislation dealing with alternative medicine. Only a handful of members of Congress have shown much interest in the topic. What is striking about them is that their politics vary widely. Some, like Orrin Hatch, are well-known conservatives. Their support of freedom of choice for therapy is compatible with a longstanding antipathy toward most regulatory policies, including restrictions on the rights of citizens to own guns or on corporations to pollute the environment. But others are Democrats, some quite liberal, who generally support regulation and the involvement of the federal government in the health care system. These liberal politicians often trace their support for alternative medicine to personal experiences that convinced them conventional medicine was too limited in some way. Jim Moran, a Virginia Democrat, has spoken and written movingly of the choices he and his wife faced when their three-year-old daughter was found to have a brain tumor and they were unwilling to allow radiation therapy. "Although conventional medicine provides medical miracles every day, I understand firsthand that it doesn't hold all the answers to living with a disease. Alternative medicine seeks to address health and illness within the realistic context of life and death." Moran is explicit in not calling for research to prove that alternative medicine works. He asks only that it have the same level of safety, efficacy, and cost effectiveness as mainstream care.

Tom Harkin, the Democratic senator from Iowa and an influential member of Congress, attributes the success of bee pollen in treating his severe allergies after conventional therapy failed as the key to his discovery of alternative medicine. He sees a pressing need to mainstream alternative therapies without seeking evidence that they are effective via the randomized clinical trials which federal regulatory agencies typically demand. He writes, "I know that there is something powerful here that we don't yet understand. Did I need someone to show me exactly how that was accomplished in order to experience the results I did? Of course not! And it is not necessary for the scientific community to understand the process before the American public can benefit from these therapies."

The primary sponsor of the Access to Medical Treatment Act in the House of Representatives is Peter DeFazio of Oregon, a liberal Democrat. The bill would mandate access to any treatment, FDA approved or not, as long as it had not been shown to cause harm and the patient was informed of any known risks. DeFazio wants a "holistic approach to health . . . to be part of every government agency focusing on health, especially the National Institutes of Health's National Cancer Institute and the Department of Health and Human Services."

The political support for recognizing alternative medicine within the American health care system transcends the typical Democrat-Republican distinctions. The ability of alternative medicine to bridge left and right is based on more than the fact that criticizing federal bureaucrats is one area where community oriented liberal activists and conservative business people can agree. The political right has an affinity with alternative approaches for a number of reasons beyond its affirmation of individual responsibility. Conservatives are generally in favor of protecting individual freedom of choice in most arenas. Some conservatives may favor alternative approaches because they see them as a less costly drain upon the public purse, or more likely to be paid for directly by the client. Liberals find alternative medicine compatible with their views because it calls for seeing the whole person and the social environment as factors in health. The openness of alternative approaches to empowerment and healing traditions and techniques from other cultures appeals to liberal multiculturalism. The challenge alternative medicine presents to mainstream physicians—traditionally an elite, high-income group—may also be attractive to some on the left.

Similarly, both right and left have traditional reasons to be skeptical about alternative therapies. The right would be expected to show hesitancy in attacking conventional medicine whose members and organizations have long supported the Republican party. The left has its fears about the rampant growth of alternative care as a business to accompany its concern about an overemphasis on personal responsibility for health. All these cross-currents mean that it is difficult to predict where on the political spectrum alternative medicine may draw support. As Larry Dossey told an interviewer, "Newt loves it. Bill and Hillary favor it. Who would have thought!"

The ability of alternative medicine to draw support from both sides of the political spectrum is increasingly being recognized by advocates and practitioners. Given the diverse base of political support, the most important political battle it faces is the simple act of being recognized as a cohesive entity. The basic nature of this matter makes it relatively easy for many different types of practitioners, who usually disagree on many matters, to see that they need to present a unified front. The specific form of alternative medicine cannot take shape until there is a general perception of alternative medicine as a cohesive enterprise. With the exception of a handful of extremists, building this cohesion has become the most pressing political goal of those involved in alternative medicine.

The Office of Alternative Medicine (OAM)

By the early 1990s the interest in alternative medicine on the part of the public, politicians, and the existing health professionals had greatly increased. The media was constantly posing questions about alternative medicine: What are the clinical outcomes to alternative therapies? Can alternative approaches be integrated into conventional medical settings, and carried out by mainstream providers? How cost effective is alternative care? How can alternative practitioners be best trained and certified? Yet reliable answers were almost impossible to find. The federal government had already taken on, de facto, much of the task of answering similar questions about conventional care, largely through the work and grants of the National Institutes of Health. It did not seem unreasonable that the government, and the NIH, along with other agencies, might play a similar role in terms of alternative medicine.

Berkley Bedell, a former Iowa congressman who believed that alternative therapies cured his prostate cancer and Lyme disease, had long envisioned that the NIH should be doing much more to evaluate and promote such treatments. Bedell's close friend, Senator Tom Harkin, was head of the Senate committee that oversaw the NIH budget. After bee pollen cured Harkin's own allergies, Bedell was able to convince him to have the Appropriations Committee declare that it was dissatisfied with NIH's approach to alternative care and provide $2 million as start-up funds for an office "to fully investigate and validate these practices."

NIH responded to the demand from the Appropriations Committee in the same way that it had dealt with other politically mandated responsibilities; it created a program office called the Office of Alternative Medicine within the Office of the Director. This was not the first program office to be established at the NIH. The first of such offices, the Office of Disease Prevention, was formed in 1985 after Congress complained that little NIH funding went toward understanding how to prevent, as opposed to how to treat, disease. Within a decade, eight such offices had been formed related to rare diseases, AIDS, women's health, minority health, dietary supplements, behavioral sciences, disease prevention, and alternative medicine. With the exception of the AIDS office, none have "any central control over the distribution of any research funds, but they do co-fund some projects and supplement existing grant programs." With little money, and even less bureaucratic leeway, it is no surprise that the special offices are frequently seen as political intrusions on "real science" and a sop to the scientifically uninformed politicians who control NIH funding.

The brief history of the Office of Alternative Medicine has been particularly stormy. In October 1992, the OAM got its first director, Joseph Jacobs, a Yale-trained pediatrician. He was beleaguered from all sides from the start. NIH insiders and critics of the very idea of OAM claimed he was bureaucratically inept and too demanding for the office. Jacobs felt his NIH colleagues had "the limited view of the world that specialists have" and was surprised to find that the world-renowned NIH clinical facilities didn't offer any sort of primary care. NIH understood illness only through specialization and subspecialization.

Jacobs received minimal support from advocates of alternative practice, some of whom served on OAM's advisory board. They felt he was too mainstream, too eager to please the NIH director, and too committed to rigorous scientific evaluation of alternative therapies, with the goal of merging them into conventional care. Berkley Bedell harshly criticized Jacobs for his commitment to clinical trials of alternative therapies. Instead, Bedell called for nonrandom field studies that could simply "validate" alternative techniques by documenting that people who used them reported success. Some members of the advisory board felt that following the traditional NIH pattern of giving grants to academic researchers through a competitive process was just a waste of time. The *New York Times* described the gulf between the mainstream of NIH and OAM as "so profound that it will require a magician of a new director to solve it."

Jacobs insisted on following the typical NIH protocol. He solicited grant proposals and got 452 back for a first round of minuscule ($30,000) awards. The Division of Research Grants, not OAM, assembled panels of reviewers and eventually allocated thirty grants. I received one grant to study the experiences of people who use homeopathy. The initial total level of funding was itself "homeopathic"; the $2 million OAM received was about one five ten-thousandth (0.0005 percent) of the total NIH budget. Despite awarding the grants, and an additional appropriation of $1.8 million for alternative medicine center grants, OAM rapidly fell into chaos.

Twenty months after taking office, Jacobs resigned with a "blast" at both politicians like Harkin, who were OAM's major supporters, and at the independent OAM advisory council. Jacobs's major complaint was that neither the politicians nor the council members, who largely represented alternative practitioners and users, were willing to support true scientific analysis of alternative therapies. Nor were they committed to Jacobs's goal of integrating alternative therapies into mainstream medical institutions through "cooperative centers." Instead, he claimed that Harkin and others were attempting to "micromanage" the office by insisting that it fund specific projects such as Burzynski's antineoplasm research on cancer and field studies that could illustrate how many people were satisfied with various alternative therapies. Jacobs said, "I wouldn't trust what comes out of my office under a system like that." He supported those like David Eisenberg, the Harvard physician who wrote a widely cited study of the utilization of alternative medicine. Eisenberg testified to Congress at a contentious June 1993 hearing that OAM should do "unbiased studies . . . by people who have no vested interest." Harkin and others saw this as a blatant attempt to divert OAM funds to established universities.

The bad feelings heightened on both sides when Jacobs learned that the OAM staff had gone along with demands from Harkin's office and included four anti-Jacobs activists on an OAM advisory committee. The advisory committee, in turn, criticized Jacobs when it learned that some large OAM center grants had gone to those like Eisenberg who had supported the idea of funding centers and had been given early drafts of the grant solicitation. Many alternative providers criticized this bias toward "insiders" as the most flagrant form of the "credentialist" stance of OAM, which essentially froze out true alternative healers from OAM money and insured equivocal findings about outcomes.

Jacobs was replaced by Alan Trachtenberg, a physician who was also trained in acupuncture and homeopathy, as acting director of OAM. Trachtenberg served from October 1994 until July 1995 when the current director, Wayne Jonas, took over. Also a physician, Jonas came to OAM after doing laboratory research in toxicology and immunology at the Walter Reed Army Institute of Research where he was a lieutenant colonel. He had worked for the Surgeon General's Office as well as on other government health projects and was sophisticated about the ways of the federal government. He immediately undertook a major staff reorganization and adopted a less rigid position on research. His guiding principle was that research should be "scientifically rigorous and contextually sensitive." In practice this meant defining effectiveness "in the context of the patient who receives the therapy. . . . Patient preferences and the subjective experience should be considered. . . . Research models are needed that capture the global and long-term outcomes. . . ." Jonas decreed that OAM would develop partnerships with a broader array of nonacademic organizations as well as universities.

Jonas's stance had an immediate positive effect on morale

and relations with the alternative medical community. Gar Hildenbrand, one of the anti-Jacobs members of the advisory committee, sought "to make up for lost time" and felt that "we are now at a time when the Office has no controversy. I am extraordinarily optimistic." Jonas's more flexible stance has borne its share of criticisms. It was attacked in a series of front-page *New York Times* articles. The headline of one piece—"In Quests Outside Mainstream, Medical Projects Rewrite Rules"—set the tone. OAM's grant standards were termed "questionable" and "dubious." The credentials of "most of the researchers who have received funding from the office" were called into question for their lack of "a track record," and the very existence of the office was derided as a mere political necessity. (When asked why the OAM had been created, Dr. Bernadine Healy, the head of the NIH at the time, said "We had no choice.") The article cited critics who challenged the entire grant review process ("If the reviews had been conducted strictly by scientists, probably nothing would have been funded") and concluded that "to critics . . . the most troubling aspect of the Office of Alternative Medicine is that its very existence lends an air of scientific credibility to treatments that most scientists would disavow." This last quote in the article came from Ursula Goodenough, a biologist at Washington University in St. Louis. She had co-authored an op-ed piece entitled "Buying Snake Oil With Tax Dollars: Why is the NIH Touting Alternative Medicine?" in the *New York Times* a few months earlier that laid out the arguments later elaborated upon in the news story. Goodenough had asked, "Should there be an Office of Alternative Medicine to evaluate unconventional practices? Not one that elevates magical notions to matters of serious scientific debate."

Both Joe Jacobs and Wayne Jonas responded to the op-ed article with letters pointing out that OAM does not "tout" any specific therapy, noting that "alternative medicine is not all quackery and not all quacks are alternative medical practitioners," and generally decrying the politicization of the OAM and its task. In actuality the politicization of OAM was already well established by that time. Writing in *Alternative Therapies,* Representative John Porter of Illinois told the alternative medical community that the "only" way to preserve OAM funding, no less increase it, would be through heightened political action and lobbying. "To be successful, you must get to know your congressman and establish the personal bonds of trust and respect that come from a relationship that develops through many contacts over time. Only by continual insistence by a large group of patients and practitioners can a cause such as alternative medicine be ensured a strong voice in the budgetary process."

Regardless of the controversy surrounding the creation of the OAM and its internal problems, there can be no question that its formation represents a major political triumph for alternative medicine. Critics like Park and Goodenough are correct. The real issue is not any specific decision or research OAM conducts. The very existence of OAM implies an overall stamp of approval about what knowledge is officially accepted as legitimate or "real." The ongoing existence of OAM represents the U.S. government's acceptance, at least on a preliminary level, of a set of ideas that the established health professions have actively resisted for many years. Whereas the conventional view has been that the use of alternative medicine is an irrational act, usually undertaken by uninformed and desperate people, the creation and activities of OAM indicates that the government no longer automatically or uncritically accepts this view. Even more fundamental is that OAM's existence undercuts the belief that the existing health professions, and the institutions they control, are the only environment in which valid diagnosis, treatment, and healing can occur. If OAM exists and grows, the very nature of what is rational and what is irrational with regard to health and illness is brought into question. This is why OAM, despite its tiny budget, has attracted the wrath of many mainstream scientists and physicians. Their response reflects their fear of losing their power and legitimacy to the demands for recognition and political power by advocates of alternative medicine. After all, mainstream medicine has had a near monopoly on the definitions that alternative medicine questions. OAM simultaneously provides a structure for initiating the legitimization of these alternative views and for promoting them in a wide range of settings.

In the past few years, OAM's presence has begun to be felt on matters beyond simply the conceptual acceptance of a new paradigm of health. Other parts of the health bureaucracy have begun to show the first signs of accepting the legitimacy of alternative medicine. In 1996, the federal advisory panel on AIDS research issued a highly critical report on the success of government funding policies and priorities over the coming years. One of the recommendations of this group of highly regarded scientists was to call for an examination of what alternative medicine had to offer. OAM itself has begun to work jointly with other parts of NIH to cosponsor meetings, working groups, and conferences on this and other topics. The Conference on Behavioral Medicine and Relaxation Techniques in October of 1995 is typical. After conducting a technical assessment, this group concluded that these approaches should be integrated into standard medical treatments for chronic pain and insomnia. A summary paper encouraging this integration was published a few months later in the *Journal of the American Medical Association*. OAM was also able to prevail on the FDA to reclassify acupuncture needles for general medical use. Until that time (1995), these needles were considered "investigational" and technically illegal to use except as part of a research protocol. OAM was instrumental in using acupuncture's new normalized status to justify making treatment reimbursable under Medicare.

In 1996, OAM made its first foray into the direct provision of health care services. The research center it funds at Bastyr University, an accredited school of naturopathic medicine outside of Seattle, began to manage the nation's first publicly-funded natural medical clinic. The largely Republican Metro-politan King County council unanimously approved establishing the clinic in early 1995. News accounts described the personal past experiences of some council members dealing with their own prostate cancer as decisive in their support for the center. The center offers conventional medical services along with referrals for a wide range of alternative therapies on site. OAM's most direct involvement in the program is through the research study it has built to evaluate client satisfaction, cost-effectiveness, and health outcomes.

Currently, OAM survives as an ongoing and growing agency within the federal health bureaucracy. Over a period when the NIH budget has remained at a steady state, OAM's budget appropriation has increased to $7.4 million in FY 1996 and $12 million in FY 1997. In 1997, OAM was designated Collaborating Center for the study of traditional medicine by The World Health Organization. Its Database and Evaluation Section currently respond to thousands of queries each year, and its research program is growing, in part through linkages with other parts of NIH. In the fall of 1998, OAM's congressional supporters prevailed on the NIH to upgrade it from a "program office" to a full "center" with control over its own $50 million budget.

The creation and continuing growth of OAM represents a political triumph for alternative medicine in its ability to transcend the usual liberal-conservative political boundaries. An increased reliance on personal responsibility, skepticism about the efficacy of high tech and highly professionalized interventions, and a renewed emphasis on volunteerism and other community-based interventions are all themes that can appeal to those on both the right and the left. Each theme is well ensconced within the values and approaches comprising alternative medicine. The convergence of these trends within alternative medicine makes it likely that, regardless of the vehemence of its critics, OAM will survive and grow over the next few years.

Perhaps the greatest political impact of OAM may be on the structures and organization of alternative medicine itself. OAM's existence offers a direct political channel for alternative medicine's concerns to be heard and addressed. However, this opportunity cannot be effectively utilized if alternative medicine is faction ridden, or heavily influenced by its most extreme elements. The existence of OAM puts strong pressure on the alternative medical community to build consensus on issues such as educational standards, certification requirements, licensure, research protocols, and relationships with conventional providers. What is unclear thus far is how the leadership of alternative medicine will respond to this opportunity. The history of medicine, as well as that of other professions, indicates that if alternative medicine is to seize upon these opportunities, some elite group must emerge to offer a vision of the future. In the case of alternative medicine, the basic concepts that underlie that vision are not as much at issue as the structural manifestations of these ideas. OAM's ability to offer alternative medicine a "carrot" in terms of societal legitimacy, intellectual acceptance, and financial stability may have the potential to be a decisive factor in the future.

Regardless of its conceptual affinities with a variety of strong political views, the actual politics of alternative medicine are moderate and its political goals modest. The political concerns of alternative medicine lie in achieving recognition through the time-honored means of licensure, accreditation, and recognition by the state. Inevitably, such goals lead to moderation, accommodation, and compromise, rather than extremism in any form. Those who hold extreme views are likely to find themselves increasingly marginalized in the future. It may well be true that the increasing merging of alternative medicine, with its emphasis on personal responsibility, into conventional settings helps to foster and reinforce a climate of diminishing expectations. But, as will be demonstrated in the next chapter, this atmosphere permeates the medical mainstream and can hardly be blamed on alternative therapies.

7 Alternative Medicine, Mainstream Markets

Healers in every society have been compensated for their work. In America doctors have made a good living, at least since 1910 when the Flexner Report sharply restricted the number of new physicians. Until very recently, the medical profession has exemplified how one group can create, control, and monopolize a market for its own economic gains. But as centralization, bureaucratization, and corporate control of health care have rapidly advanced in the decades since the 1960s, the marketplace has reshaped the form and practice of American medicine. The term "nonprofit" is less and less likely to characterize hospitals and other health care organizations. Today, while the economic power of physicians as a group has declined somewhat, the practice of medicine is more responsive to economic forces than at any time in our nation's history. It is within this emerging but extremely powerful pattern of proprietary corporate dominance of medical care that alternative medicine must be viewed.

Americans spend a large amount of money on alternative medicine. Based on one widely cited study, an estimated $21.2 *billion* were spent on payments to alternative providers alone in 1997. Vitamin supplements, herbs, books, and other supplemental costs brought the total up to $27 billion. Since these figures were derived from estimates of visits for treatment, not preventive services, they are likely to underestimate the actual size of the nation's expenditures on alternative providers and therapies. These figures are about equal to the amount Americans spend out-of-pocket on hospital care, and twice the amount spent for out-of-pocket physician's fees. It is undeniable that a lot of money is being spent on alternative medicine in our society.

Alternative Medicine as Small Business

Until the 1980s, the economic aspects of alternative healing, to the extent they were portrayed at all in journalistic or academic accounts, consisted of single practitioners in fee-for-service practices. In this fundamental regard, the economic organization of both conventional and alternative practitioners has been quite similar. Some accounts emphasized the unregulated entrepreneurial dimensions of these alternative practices, while others stressed the difficulties inherent in running a small, if deviant, business. Today, with the growing prominence of alternative therapies, and the growth of specialty publications, direct mail advertising, the Internet, and many other sources of information, it is very easy to find an immense range of alternative practitioners who operate as classic entrepreneurial small business people by offering their knowledge, skills, and products to the public.

In large part, such practitioners operate self-consciously as business people. Their claims of therapeutic efficacy, safety, product purity, and credentials are largely unevaluated. In some cases their goals and honesty are above reproach. In other instances, the practitioners might more accurately be described as "hucksters" or "medicine men" whose only goal is to maximize their own incomes. Their methods may seem highly questionable. The ELF bracelet to counter the impact of low frequency radiation that emanates from AC electric current is promoted as "highly effective" for alleviating chronic arthritis, fatigue, and back pain, as well as improving alertness and vision. The mail order price is $39. Or you can resist this same list of ailments, along with allergies and insomnia, by purchasing mattresses filled with magnets. The manufacturer cites research on 431 people to back up the claim that "in the search for a universal cure-all, none fits the description nearly as well as magnetic energy therapy." A queen size mattress has 364 magnets, while the king size has 468.

Alternative health and medicine fairs such as the Whole Life Expo, which attracts thousands of paying visitors in many large cities, are open to essentially any exhibitor who is willing to pay for space. A "natural sex" booth offered homeopathic aphrodisiacs, and trampolines ("jumping for health") are sold as a possible treatment for cancer as well as a good way to burn calories. Products like aloe vera gel are promoted as cures for every imaginable problem. One manufacturer distributes literature offering aloe vera as a cure for so many illnesses and conditions that they are simply grouped by their first letter; for example, "C: cancer, candida, corneal ulcers, contusions, canker sores, cold sores, cuts, cataracts, chapped and chafed skin and lips, coughs, colds, colitis, carbuncles, colic, cradle cap, cystitis, chemotherapy, constipation." Cell Tech, a producer of "super blue green algae," sells its product for a similar array of problems, along with the additional possibility that it may raise one's I.Q. up to twenty points. Vendors present all sorts of products as having restorative or health promoting powers. Neon lights in free-form sculpture that reduce flicker and glare (the basic unit costs $600) are marketed as essential for health as a good diet. A professional artist sells portraits as "Heal Thy Self—Journey Portraits" that can "be an integral part in the making and healing of the self."

Sometimes these products are aggressively marketed through "pyramids." Juice from the Hawaiian noni fruit is widely offered as an aid in treating cancer, diabetes, chronic pain, sinusitis, addictions, arthritis, and many other problems. One of the major distributors charges $40 for a month's supply of juice. But if you purchase a four-month supply, you become a "distributor" and are charged $30. The more you buy and resell to others, the less the cost. The company describes this as "a compensation plan that will set the standard for the industry for decades to come."

Around the nation, scores of alternative healers have established their own centers, publish newsletters, maintain websites, and offer every imaginable sort of training and therapy. The School for Enlightenment and Healing, run by Michael Mamas in San Diego, offers year-long coursework (approximately one hundred hours of class plus twelve hours of personal healing for $2,000), or weekend workshops to develop proficiency in "meditation, channeling, subtle perception, esoteric knowledge of consciousness, psychodynamics, long distance and telephone healing, past life healing, and body scanning." In many larger metropolitan areas there are now directories such as *The Healthy Yellow Pages,* which describes itself as a directory for "environmentally and socially responsible resources, health, fitness, and bodywork, natural foods markets and restaurants, natural remedies and products, and counseling, education, and spiritual resources." The 1996 edition for the Los Angeles region has listings in hundreds of categories. Glancing at the titles under the "A" section gives some sense of the range: acupressure, acupuncture, addiction recovery-treatment services and support, AIDS and HIV services and support, air purifiers and filtering, Alexander Technique, alien-UFO abductee support, allergy treatment, alternative energy, angel artwork and gifts, animal healers, animal humane and ethical treatment organizations, anti-aging products and services, appliance and metal recycling, applied kinesiology, aromatherapy, artists, astrology, attorneys, aura and chakra services, Ayurvedic medicine. The *New Age Journal* puts out an annual 200-page nationwide directory of these services. Among its listings in the 1995–1996 issue were twenty-one different "natural healing therapies," eighteen "movement therapies," fifteen "energy techniques," thirty-one "bodywork and massage therapies," and twenty-eight types of counseling techniques. Each is presented as uncritically as any listing in the phone book.

Some alternative medical organizations have grown to the extent that they no longer need to rely on directories or referral services to get clients. The Cancer Control Society, based in southern California, now promotes a range of alternative therapies for cancer, AIDS, and other degenerative diseases. It is intimately tied to a group of seven clinics in Tijuana, Mexico, such as the Stella Maris clinic and Oasis Hospital. To critics, these clinics have epitomized medical quackery and the exploitation of the desperately ill. Their location in Mexico, just over the border from San Diego, has liberated them from American laws and regulations while affording them easy access to a vast supply of clients. Despite its marginal status, the Cancer Control Society has expanded tremendously as a "nonprofit educational and charitable organization" that holds well-attended conventions and offers California-approved continuing education credit for nurses who take its programs on nontoxic cancer therapies.

Each of the clinics associated with the Cancer Control Society has its own individualized approach to treatment. Perhaps the most widely known is Laetrile, a nontoxic substance that is administered with an array of vitamins and enzymes to improve immune functioning and produce antibodies to fight tumors. Similar claims are made for many other substances: Hoxsey therapy, hydrazine sulfate, Issel's Whole Body therapy, Kelley's Nutritional metabolic therapy, shark cartilage, Livingston therapy, Revici Therapy, etc. Each has its own advocates and clinics.

Better known than most, but typical in its claims and presentation, is the Gerson Clinic, which describes itself as "curing incurables." Max Gerson was a physician, who in the 1930s announced that adhering to a strict diet had cured his migraines. Gerson went on to claim great success using diet to treat TB, diabetes (Albert Schweitzer was one of his successes), and later, cancer. The treatment consists of a strict very low salt vegetarian diet supplemented by ten servings a day of freshly crushed fruit. A patient consumes the nutrients from twenty pounds a day of organic food, augmented by at least three coffee enemas to rid the body of toxins. Advocates promote the regimen as capable of preventing almost any incurable disease if it is "followed diligently." For those who are already ill, the promises are somewhat more subdued. Yet, the Gerson Clinic put out literature offering many examples of people with a wide array of incurable and often fatal conditions who have been totally cured. One brochure reads, "Pancreas cancer and liver cancers have no record in the world in all of medical history of being cured . . . two cases shown here are cured . . . lung cancer . . . ten such cases . . . three cases of hopeless melanoma recoveries . . . thousands of people cured of other 'incurable' diseases . . . high blood pressure seldom lasts more than 4 days after beginning treatment . . . ." In addition to its clinic in Tijuana, the Gerson Institute offers a nationwide series of courses, books, and tapes on its therapies. Objective financial information about the Gerson Clinic and similar clinics are very difficult to obtain. But it is clear that information about them is very readily available to the public. It is likely that their recognition, popularity, and financial success are higher than they were a few decades ago.

Regardless of their therapeutic efficacy, the sorts of clinics, products, and practitioners described above represent one dimension of the organizational and economic reality of alternative medicine: independent, fee for service/product, capitalism. Their needs and desires are the same as those of most small businesses and entrepreneurs: to be left alone. Regulation of any sort is anathema to them. They see the government, insurance companies, and regulatory agencies such as the FDA, state medical boards, pharmaceutical companies, and most conventional practitioners as allied against them. They, and their adherents and supporters, often equate the phrase "freedom of medical choice" with the freedom of practitioners and consumers to utilize any therapy they wish. These providers and organizations, along with many of their clients, embody and reflect the values of laissez-faire capitalism in its most extreme form. A few decades ago their immersion in these economic beliefs would not have differentiated them from conventional practitioners. But today, their rejection of all forms of regulation from both within and outside the profession set them far apart.

Although alternative practitioners traditionally shared much of the same economic motivation as conventional physicians, in one other key respect they remained very distinct. Well prior to the advent of "managed care," mainstream doctors were tied to the corporate world through their reliance on drug and medical equipment manufacturers and insurance companies. These links deepened as the corporate world began to fund medical research and medical schools, and became omnipresent in the processes through which medicine gained its political power and autonomy. In contrast, alternative practitioners were almost totally excluded from any contact with the corporate world. Today, the barriers between alternative medicine and America's large corporations have begun to crumble.

Alternative Medicine as Big Business

One reason for this change has been that alternative techniques have become so popular large corporations have begun to view them as a significant source of revenue. Deepak Chopra's books and tapes (audio and video) have been phenomenally successful. His book *Ageless Body, Timeless Mind* has sold over seven million copies. Chopra's lectures earn him $25,000 each, and he is beginning to write screenplays for production by major studios. Chopra has his own clinic in San Diego, a firm (Infinite Possibilities) to market his workshops, a line of herbal products (OptiCalm, OptiEnergy), and agreements to develop music CDs, as well as his own monthly magazine (*Deepak Chopra's Infinite Possibilities for Body, Mind, and Soul*). The magazine's subscription solicitation offers the possibility of, "perfection in health . . . abundance of love . . . overflowing creativity . . . integrity on the job . . . ever increasing vitality . . . expansion of consciousness . . . affluence and generosity . . . playfulness and joy . . . and a long, long life to enjoy it all." Chopra has published seventeen books since 1985. His most recent titles were brought out by Crown / Harmony Books, an imprint of Random House, which is the largest English language trade publisher.

With their economic muscle, Chopra's books receive massive publicity and he receives best placement at the corporate owned bookstores like Borders and Barnes and Noble. The popularity of Chopra's work led to his appearance on the covers of both *Newsweek* and *Time*. This in turn increased his popularity even more and most likely boosted sales of his work, including the Time Life videos. The precise impact of this success on Chopra's work is difficult to assess. But his reduced emphasis on Indian religion and increasing reliance on Western religious sources (see Chapter 4) make his work more marketable to a mass American audience. Does this change make his work more appealing to a large publisher? Or does having a large publisher who is willing to heavily promote his work make Chopra more willing to shift its focus? All that can be said with assurance is that there is an affinity between the accessibility of Chopra's more recent work and the mass marketing goals of Random House and Time Life. The day after Chopra appeared for a full hour on Oprah Winfrey's television show, *Ageless Body, Timeless Mind* sold 137,000 copies. Many authors and publishers would be well aware that appearing on "Oprah" has the potential to greatly influence sales. They also know that the Oprah Winfrey show seeks guests who can offer viewers an appealing personality, combined with a story of personal struggle that leads to a life-transforming message. Chopra has all this, plus products to market. It's a potentially ideal fit. The question is: Does the medium alter the message?

The work of Andrew Weil provides another example of how large corporations are beginning to assume a dominant role in the marketing of information about alternative medicine. Weil is the author of a number of very successful books about alternative medicine. He currently resides in Arizona where he is assembling a program for physicians at the University of Arizona Medical School, which he hopes to turn into a residency program in complementary therapy. Weil also created an immensely popular website on the Internet that receives almost 85,000 hits every day. Every weekday Weil answers a reader's question, offers links to all sorts of related sites and resources, and makes available archives of his previous responses and the basic content of many of his books. In mid-1997, the website, which had long carried some advertising banners and links, became part of the Pathfinder group, which is itself owned by Time Warner. Weil's message now literally comes wrapped in a listing of other Time Warner websites. In September of 1997 Weil reorganized and enlarged his website. Among the new features are links to commercial sites, including a service for purchasing the vitamins Weil suggests (the site will customize the needs of each visitor) as well as a direct link to Barnes and Noble to order the books (his own and others) he recommends. *Time Magazine* ran a cover story on Weil just a few weeks before its parent company took over his website.

The examples of Weil and Chopra are significant for what they tell us about the changing relationship of alternative medicine and elite American corporations. The latter now view alternative medicine as fully legitimate content for the mass market and a good source of profit for themselves, regardless of the validity of the message they offer. The major Time Warner publications, *Fortune, Money Magazine,* and others, are all linked to Weil's Pathfinder website. The overarching message to the public is that Time Warner's business is helping you improve the quality of your life by doing such things as investing for the greatest return, finding the best vacation spots, and utilizing alternative therapy. Media conglomerates are uniquely situated to help create the personalities whose products they market. The books, seminars, interviews, magazine stories, TV coverage, and infomercials all reinforce each other and generate immense revenue and profit.

Alternative medicine is fast becoming a part of "big business." Sales of homeopathic remedies reached over $100 million in 1991 and continue to grow at over 20 percent annually. Medicinal herb sales were over $1.3 billion that same year. This growth is part of a larger boom in the consumption of "natural" products of all sorts. Between 1989 and 1994, sales of organically grown fruits and vegetables almost doubled to $7.6 billion, while sales of bottled water tripled in the decade between 1984 and 1994 to almost three billion gallons. These sharply escalating figures reflect the fact that traditional sources of these products are increasing (the number of health food supermarkets of over 5,000 square feet tripled to over 650 in the three years between 1991 and 1994) as well as the fact that more mainstream retail outlets, such as most of the major drug chains, now stock lines of herbs and homeopathic remedies.

The economic trends in alternative medicine and the broader "health promotion" industry reflect the changes occurring throughout the conventional health care industry: mergers; the growing dominance of a small number of larger corporations; and the integration of previously independent producers, distributors, and clinicians into coordinated systems. Just as the growth of the conventional health care industry has encouraged large non-health care firms to enter the health care market, the rapid growth of alternative medicine has made it attractive to mainstream health and non-health corporations. For example, in the late 1960s and early 1970s, homeopathic remedies were difficult to find in most American communities. Many of them were formulated by practitioners or homeopathic pharmacies or manufactured by a few small firms. By 1991 the American market for homeopathic remedies had grown to over $100 million a year. By that time, two large European homeopathic firms had purchased smaller American companies and heavily invested in their expansion. Along with two California-based firms, they now dominate the market.

The growing market and the marketing sophistication of the revived and larger firms has led many large national drugstore chains, such as Osco/Savon and Rite-Aid, to carry homeopathic and herbal products. Most of these stores are themselves part of much larger retailing conglomerates. For example, Osco/Savon is owned by American Stores, which has begun to introduce some of the herbal remedies into its Lucky Food markets. In most cases, when one supermarket chain in a community stocks a type of product, its competitors will rapidly do the same. Thus, not only is the availability of herbal and homeopathic remedies much greater today than in the recent past, but such remedies are now accessible in entirely conventional settings. The full color advertising supplements that Osco/Savon distributes in hundreds of Sunday newspapers now include multipage promotions for herbal preparations such as ginkgo biloba ("supports mental function and memory"), Cobra for men ("powerful, all natural herbs help improve stamina, performance and pleasure"), Efalex for children ("exclusive formula . . . helps maintain eye and brain function"), and scores of similar products. Very small print at the bottom of the four pages of ads devoted to these products notes that "these statements have not been evaluated by the Food and Drug Administration. These products are not intended to diagnose, treat, cure or prevent any disease." From the vantage point of the consumer, these products have joined the mainstream. The identical pattern is evident in the sales of natural foods. Currently about 20 percent of all natural/organic foods are being sold in mass market food stores, up sharply from a few years ago when the percentage was almost nil.

Manufacturers and distributors of alternative medical products have grown increasingly sophisticated in advertising and presentation. Catalogs, mailings, websites, and promotional literature are all polished and professional. Alternative practitioners have their own "throwaway" journals such as *Healthy Answers,* filled with glossy ads, sitting in their waiting rooms. There has been a massive convergence in the form and appearance of consumer marketing of conventional and alternative medicine.

Initially, many corporations were reluctant to focus on alternative medicine since, as natural substances, vitamins, herbal remedies, and other alternative therapeutic agents could not be patented. The market has now become so big, and potentially lucrative, that big firms are increasingly drawn in. They bring an emphasis on product differentiation as a means of maximizing sales and profits. One business strategy has been to develop various combinations of vitamins and/or herbs targeted to specific problems, give them descriptive names, and sell them for well above their individual market value. A typical example of this exists in the catalog from Equinox, a direct sales firm offering "a complete line of environmentally conscious and health related products exclusively formulated to impact our lives and our planet in a positive way." This elaborate and sophisticated catalog offers hundreds of formulated products with names like "Tranquility," "Tolerance," "Super Charge," "re Charge," "Skeletal Support," "Balanced Woman," "Mind Power," etc. Each bottle of 120 capsules sells for $28, which is, conservatively, three to four times the cost of the same substances purchased individually.

A visit to a health food or large drug store will reveal large variations in price for most alternative remedies. A substance like melatonin can vary in cost by up to 300 percent for equal dosages. This variability in cost means that manufacturers have to find some way to make their products seem unique, in order to justify higher prices. When melatonin was a rare specialty item, such cost differences meant little to a manufacturer. However, since 1994, when melatonin suddenly became popular as a "cure" for scores of problems, and the subject of a cover story in *Newsweek,* many millions of bottles have been sold each year. Since that time, the ability to command even small price differences could result in a significant gain for a manufacturer or distributor.

The marketing of herbs is considerably more complicated than that of vitamins. Vitamins have long been sold in the United States and are held up to clear regulatory standards by the FDA, independent of their efficacy in treating any condition. Vitamin C may or may not reduce your probability of catching a cold. But, when you buy vitamin C you can be confident that the substance in the pill is vitamin C, at the dosage stated on the bottle. Equivalent standards for herbs do not exist, and there have already been a number of exposés of firms marketing ginseng and other herbal products in capsules containing none of the product in question. In the United States, the market for medicinal herbs was $1.27 billion in 1995, and is increasing by over 10 percent a year. The worldwide market for medicinal herbs was over $60 billion that same year. In this country, ten herbs (echinacea, garlic, goldenseal, ginseng, ginkgo biloba, saw palmetto, aloe, ephedra, Siberian ginseng, and cranberry) account for over half of all sales. Competition to present herbal products as genuine is fierce, as it is believed that buyers will pay vastly higher prices for something they are confident is pure.

With its reputation as an enhancer of overall immune functioning and sexual prowess, ginseng has become quite popular. Many American consumers assume that the herb's long popularity in Asia means that Korean or Siberian ginseng connotes high quality. In fact, ginseng grown in Wisconsin is acknowledged to be the most powerful and costly. But when the economic crisis of 1998 decimated the Asian market, prices for Wisconsin ginseng plunged by up to 85 percent. Now American growers are faced with pressure to create a brand-name consciousness for their high priced roots and seeds in the domestic market. To fend off cheaper imports from Asia and Canada, Wisconsin growers have consolidated and formed joint marketing campaigns using a seal of authenticity for "genuine Wisconsin ginseng." Meanwhile, PharmaPrint, a California firm, is one of a number of companies attempting to isolate the active ingredients in ginseng and many other herbs in order to synthesize them. This will make the product patentable and saleable at a very high premium.

Herbs are increasingly part of a rapidly growing organic food industry (over 20 percent yearly since 1990) that is also undergoing consolidation. Firms like Whole Foods Markets have taken over a number of smaller regional markets, such as Mrs. Gooch's in California. In 1996 Whole Foods, based in Texas, merged with Fresh Fields of New Jersey. It rapidly took over two other regional health food chains, Bread and Circus in Massachusetts and The Merchant of Vino in Michigan, yielding a chain of seventy-six organic food "superstores" in seventeen states with annual sales of over $750 million. The following year, the company's stock rose 240 percent. Also in 1996, the two next largest chains, Alfalfa's and Wild Oats, merged to create a chain of forty-nine stores. Together these chains sell almost 20 percent of all the "natural/organic" food in the nation. Each of these chains presents itself to the public as a "complete" market, meaning that it stocks items such as Häagen-Dazs ice cream and Cheerios, which many would be hard pressed to define as "natural" or "health" food. Although purists see this as the organic food industry "selling out" in order to get more mainstream customers, it is also a reflection of the way in which "health food," herbal medicine, and conventional food marketing are intersecting. Large supermarkets stock herbs and organic produce, while large "health food" stores sell Haagen Daz. This convergence—which is driven and abetted from both sides by a need to maximize profit, match competition, and increase market share—may foreshadow developments in the availability of clinical health services.

The confluence of the organic and mainstream consumer can be appreciated by looking at a recent issue of *Prevention* magazine, the flagship publication of Rodale Press. Started in 1950, *Prevention* has probably done more to encourage the consumption of natural foods and herbs for health purposes than any other single source in the United States. The lead story of the April 1997 issue, entitled "The PMS Herb," promotes black cohash root as the most effective way to deal with premenstrual symptoms. This issue contains advertising from Lever Brothers, Folgers Coffee, The National Milk Board, Dupont, Schering (for Claritan, a prescription medication), Mars Candy (Three Musketeers Bars), Ford, and at least a dozen other national consumer companies. The Rodale Press advertising kit for *Prevention* claims an audited circulation of 3.25 million copies with a readership of over 11 million. The reader's median income is given as $38,864 per household, with 57.1 percent of readers having at least some college education. National corporations are well aware of the fact that the market for alternative medical consumer products is the same market as that for most upscale consumer products.

The Convergence into Mainstream Health Care

The impressive growth of alternative medicine as an independent economic entity is only one aspect of the overall picture. The rapidly increasing integration of alternative medicine into conventional medicine's organizations and economic reality is, overall, a much more significant development. The growing organizational and financial convergence between alternative and mainstream medicine developed within the context of vast changes occurring in mainstream medicine over the past two decades. At the most basic level these changes themselves arose out of growing consumer dissatisfaction with the cost and efficacy of conventional medicine; a similar array of factors underlie the public's enhanced receptivity to alternative approaches.

One fundamental factor underlying this dissatisfaction arises from the changing demographic composition of American society. As the population ages, morbidity and mortality are increasingly attributed to chronic disease. Chronic illness is typically related to lifestyle patterns and is marked by long-term degeneration of the individual's ability to function socially as well as biologically. Behavioral and psychological factors are often important in the cause, course, and efficacy of therapy in chronic conditions. It is just such conditions that conventional medical science has been least effective in controlling and upon which alternative approaches claim to have their greatest impact.

Policymakers and planners have generally responded to these demographic and epidemiologic changes by calling for health policies to prevent or delay the onset of chronic illness and lower the cost of care associated with chronic illness. In particular, they tend to view "high tech" medical interventions for dealing with the burden of ongoing chronic illness as too costly and often ineffective. A 1996 report in *JAMA* claimed that by the year 2030, 148 million Americans would suffer from at least one chronic condition. The authors estimate that the total cost of health care in that year will be $798 billion, as opposed to 659 billion in 1996. A common response to this ballooning expense has been to emphasize the use of primary care providers, as opposed to specialists, for the care of chronic illness.

In addition, policymakers recognize that many people are dissatisfied with the care they or their loved ones receive when they have a chronic illness. Patients frequently have too little "choice and voice" in their own care, a problem heightened by the rapidly growing cultural diversity within the population.

Patients' sense that their physician genuinely cares for them and will truly act in their best interest increasingly conflicts with the emerging nature of medical practice. This is reflected by the finding that a majority of people leave their physician's office unsatisfied with the visit due to the nature of the interaction with the doctor.

While the genesis and documentation of these criticisms of conventional care are independent of alternative medicine, their acceptance carries an elective affinity to alternative approaches. Indeed, the widespread acceptance of these criticisms and policy objectives among politicians was one of the primary reasons for the founding of OAM.

Over the past two decades, the American health care system has undergone a major set of interrelated changes in response to the factors I've described above. While unplanned in any systematic sense, insurance companies, large employers, and the federal government (via Medicare), have brought about three major changes in the organization of medical care services:

1. A rapid increase in for-profit large corporate chain ownership of every type of health care organization. This includes a rising number of mergers, acquisitions, and diversifications among hospitals, nursing homes, immediate and emergency care facilities, hospital supply companies, mental health and substance abuse centers, health maintenance organizations, home health care services, and hospital management systems. Currently, corporate chains own more than 15 percent of all U.S. hospitals, and the number is rapidly growing. This does not include the large number of nonprofit hospitals that have turned their management over to corporate entities.
2. Managed care has become the dominant way in which more and more people receive their conventional medical care. This vaguely defined term means

that care is monitored on the basis of whether it is truly "necessary" according to criteria predefined by someone other than the attending physician. Such care is often paid for by a capitation system in which a set amount of money is allocated in advance for each patient. Thus, practitioners are very conscious of how much their care will cost, as well as the consequences to themselves or their colleagues if that amount is exceeded. In some managed care plans, spending less per patient results in higher profits for the corporation and bonuses for the physician. By the end of 1997, over 90 percent of physicians in private practice had contracted with at least one managed care plan.

3. Health care organizations have become increasingly specialized and diverse. Free-standing emergency centers, separate from hospitals, are common. Specialists, such as fertility experts or opthamologists, work together and contract to provide their services to other groups of physicians or health maintenance organizations in so-called "carve outs."

Separately and together these changes mean that economic efficiency and profit making have become key determinants in how health care is organized and how providers use specific therapies. Ironically, it is this very emphasis on reducing costs, building market share, and producing profit that has made the current system more hospitable to alternative medicine. Almost without exception, the modalities of alternative medicine are relatively inexpensive to administer. They usually take place outside of the hospital and do not require much in the way of high-tech equipment. Most alternative approaches emphasize prevention and improved functioning as opposed to a cure. The non-Western origin of many alternative approaches is especially appealing to immigrant groups and others, which makes them good marketing devices for attracting customers. The pervasive emphasis on individual responsibility for one's own health and healing tends to diminish dependence on professionals. For all these reasons, the new corporate managed care enterprises have become more open to integrating alternative medicine into their organizations.

The current status of most forms of alternative medicine (chiropractic is an exception) makes it difficult for integration to proceed very far or fast, however. Beyond the basic issue of therapeutic efficacy of many alternative techniques, there is not very much consistency in the training, accreditation, certification, and licensure of alternative providers. In many cases this lack of credentials makes reimbursement of services difficult. An HMO can't refer a patient to a naturopathic physician if such a thing doesn't legally exist, or if the HMO has no way of knowing who is "really" trained and competent in the field. An even more basic issue is that many advocates of alternative modalities explicitly or implicitly reject integration with conventional medicine, especially in a limited or subservient role. Still, many other alternative providers feel their future economic stability is largely dependent on forging some sort of workable relationship with the medical mainstream.

Alternative Medicine as Corporate Medicine

The possibilities offered by economic integration into the medical mainstream are far more significant than the recent economic growth of alternative medicine as an encapsulated, independent entity. The amalgamation of alternative and conventional care has the potential to fundamentally alter both alternative and conventional care. As in the case of managed care that within a relatively short period of time has drastically changed the way in which physicians and hospitals behave, it is largely financial motivations, not the integration of philosophies or techniques, that have inspired the changes.

Leaders in alternative medicine commonly justify their de-

sire to integrate into mainstream medicine in terms of the supposed financial benefits that will accrue to the society as a whole,
or to particular managed care organizations. Advocates of many
alternative modalities are quick to point out the generally low
cost of their interventions, along with the high level of client
satisfaction they produce regardless of outcome. The notion
that managed care organizations which offer alternative therapies might make their clients happier by spending less money
is a powerful, if untested, incentive for HMOs and corporate
health care benefits officers. In a written debate on whether
homeopathy should be integrated into mainstream medicine,
Jennifer Jacobs, a physician and homeopath, put it this way:
"Another relevant area of research is in cost effectiveness and
outcomes. In France, research on cost-effectiveness has shown
that the annual cost to the social security system for a homeopathic physician is 15% less than that of a conventional physician and the price of the average homeopathic medicine is
one third that of standard drugs." In a similar vein, a widely
cited guide to alternative therapies offers this concluding
thought for why qigong, which is already widely used in the
United States, will be incorporated into mainstream medical
practice: "One factor makes qigong an inevitable innovation in
Western culture: the staggering cost of post-symptomatic medical intervention. With qigong, individuals learn to heal themselves and maintain their health—a profoundly cost-effective
feature."

The twenty-fifth anniversary issue of *Natural Health* magazine typified this sort of aggressive financial advocacy on the
part of the alternative community. In the article entitled "The
Medical Revolution" the author concluded:

> Perhaps the biggest momentum carrying the country toward a
> new system of health care is coming from the people who pick up
> the tab for much of the nearly one trillion dollars spent on health
> care services and products. . . . If a patient has back pain that he
> [a primary care provider] believes would improve with movement
> therapy, he'll say to the insurance representative, "look do you

want me to order an MRI for $1,200 and refer the patient to a neurosurgeon for a $20,000 laminectomy? Or do you want to pay for $350 worth of Alexander Technique? It's your choice, but I'd like you to give me your name because I plan to write the president of your company and tell him that you told me to spend $40,000 rather than $350."

The alternative community is beginning to develop alternative PPOs (preferred provider organizations) that offer conventional health plans the opportunity to form alliances with networks of alternative caregivers. They are also marketing insurance policies offering both conventional and alternative care.

The alternative community is constantly reaching out to the world of conventional medical practice, with the goal of gaining entry and further integrating alternative techniques. For example, in 1996 *Alternative Therapies* published an article by Richard Lippin, the medical director for the Atlantic Richfield Chemical Company (ARCO), which argued that alternative medicine should play an extensive role in the workplace by collaborating with the specialty of occupational medicine. Lippin believes the ability of alternative therapies to reduce stress, alleviate physical pain for problems like repetitive stress injury, and enhance productivity will yield high profits for corporations. He concluded his article with the view that it is "the desire for the United States to remain competitive in a world economy" that will bring alternative therapy into occupational medicine.

Increasingly, the medical mainstream is open to at least some integration of alternative approaches. As early as 1979, *JAMA* published an editorial entitled "Holistic Health or Holistic Hoax" which tentatively concluded that organized medicine should be more accepting of a wide range of alternative approaches. That same year the *Western Journal of Medicine* devoted an entire issue to "Orthodox Medicine, Humanistic Medicine, Holistic Medical Care." The largely positive background pieces were intended to begin a dialogue about the future relations between all three of these entities, presumed to be separate. The articles discuss the philosophy of holism and its ability to assist medicine by placing a greater emphasis on prevention and mind-body interaction, as well as on compassionate, competent care for the chronically ill. The one article that is most hesitant about the possibility of successfully integrating holistic care bases its reservations on alternative medicine's vulnerability to being co-opted. The author cautions, "But most of what is rich within the holistic orientation must necessarily remain outside a fee-for-service medical care system. And this is so because to integrate the perspective, as it translates into practice, is to erode the practice, and in turn, vitiate the perspective." Yet, it is the economic concerns that have developed since the 1979 issue of the *Western Journal of Medicine,* that have led to conventional medicine's increasing openness to alternative approaches. Managed care leadership does not necessarily believe in the efficacy of these techniques, but they hope such methods can cut costs and improve the market share of managed care organizations by boosting patient satisfaction or serving as an inducement to join.

The growth of managed care has forced conventional medicine to recognize its own limitations in effectively and efficiently (i.e., cost-effectively) dealing with chronic disease. This includes many serious, debilitating conditions like AIDS and most cancers, along with the less serious but chronic conditions such as allergies, skin problems, chronic pain, arthritis, and fatigue that fill doctors' offices. In each case mainstream medicine offers very costly therapies with little long-term efficacy. If an equally (in)effective but less costly alternative therapy could be substituted for all or part of treatment, might not at least some patients be more satisfied and overall expenditures be reduced? Combined with the growing desire to limit the overuse of many conventional therapies due to their side effects and the recognition that conventional medicine has little to offer those who wish to change their behavior or attitudes, the organizers, planners, and owners of managed care organizations see less and less reason to be resistant to alternative therapies.

This newfound openness has intensified the pressure to better answer a set of empirical questions about the quality, cost, and efficacy of alternative care: Can alternative approaches be integrated into existing managed care organizational schemes? What is the actual, as opposed to the theoretical, cost-effectiveness of the various alternative therapies? How can quality be assessed and assured? The health care industry and academic researchers have begun to address these questions. For example, for years, scores of alternative practitioners have endorsed the use of the herb St. John's wort to treat mild chronic depression, and it has even become standard medical treatment in Germany. But it wasn't until 1996 that a major medical journal published a controlled trial of St. John's wort for mild and moderate chronic depression, along with a review of the clinical literature. The trial showed the herb was almost three times as effective as a placebo, which is about the same level of improvement as offered by prescribed antidepressant drugs.

It is now common for mainstream medical journals to include cost implications in their research rationales and conclusions. Increasingly, they are extending this perspective to their empirical reports on alternative therapies. A 1995 article in the *New England Journal of Medicine* is typical. The researchers compared outcomes and costs for patients with chronic low back pain who had been seen by either primary care physicians, orthopedic surgeons, or chiropractors. They discovered almost no difference in the clinical outcomes, but found lowest cost with primary physicians and greatest client satisfaction with chiropractors. An article in the *American Journal of Hypertension* found that alternative treatments, such as relaxation and breathing exercises, can help some people reduce mild and moderate hypertension to the point of eliminating their need for medication. The authors assess the significance of their findings in terms of controlling health care costs, as much as for their impact on blood pressure. That this sort of research, rare until the mid-1990s, is becoming much more common is due not only to the efforts of alternative therapists, and OAM, but to the demands for information to serve the needs of managed care.

Academic medical centers—including Harvard, the University of California at San Francisco, and the University of Arizona—have begun programs or "centers" in alternative medicine. Regardless of the substantive concerns espoused by these organizations, economic considerations are omnipresent. Herbert Benson, head of Harvard's Mind/Body Medical Institute explained the Center's success in appealing to doctors and HMOs as "just plain money in the bank for the HMOs." The HMOs are not the only ones concerned with making a profit from alternative therapy. As is typical of many medical schools, Harvard Medical School promotes the sale of tapes from conferences run by units like the Mind/Body Institute. The complete proceedings of its 1995 "Spirituality and Healing" conference sell for $350 plus postage and handling. The tapes are marketed to physicians with a self-administered quiz worth fourteen credit hours of continuing medical education credit, as well as a "free bonus" of a thirty-six-minute videotape of conference highlights "to share with family and friends. . . . If you are not completely satisfied your money will be refunded. . . ."

In 1996, the University of California, San Francisco Medical School began its Program in Integrative Medicine to conduct research and train medical students in combining conventional and alternative treatments. Treating breast and prostate cancer as well as heart disease was the initial emphasis. Dean Ornish, the director, conducted his own "disease reversal" test of meditation, diet, and lifestyle change on heart disease. His co-director's "integrated approach" consisted of treating breast cancer with surgery, radiation, chemotherapy, meditation, yoga, and dance therapy. Ornish has been very open about promoting his methods for their financial as well as health benefits. He writes, "A primary determinant of how medicine is practiced in this country is not only science— science is important—but also what insurance pays for. . . . For every patient who goes through our program and doesn't need the surgery, somebody saves approximately $50,000." Not surprisingly, an insurance company, Mutual of Omaha, funded Ornish (and the UCSF program) to test his ideas. His pilot program, costing the firm $5,000 per person per year, was estimated to have saved treatment costs of over $7 million. Over forty insurance companies now offer at least partial reimbursement for participation in Ornish's program. A giant agribusiness firm, ConAgra, is introducing a line of prepared foods under Ornish's name.

It is clear that managed care plans' interest in alternative medicine has grown rapidly. A survey by one health care consulting firm of 156 HMOs in the ten states where HMOs have the greatest market penetration found 70 percent reported an increase in their members asking for alternative therapies to be covered in the past year. Acupuncture, chiropractic, and massage were requested most frequently. Over a third of the HMOs felt that increased coverage of alternative therapies would help their enrollment, and almost 60 percent of them indicated plans to begin or enhance their coverage of alternative therapy (especially acupuncture and chiropractic) within the next two years.

In October of 1996, Oxford Health Plans became the first large managed care company (1.4 million subscribers) to add the option of relatively comprehensive coverage for alternative medicine via a network of its own practitioners: about one thousand chiropractors, naturopaths, yoga instructors, and massage therapists, with T'ai Chi, reflexology, and other fields to be added later. Participants pay an additional 3 percent over their regular premiums. Within a few months a number of other

HMOs, such as industry giant United Health Care, had agreed to consider similar expansions, and others, like Kaiser Permanente and Lifeguard Health Care in California, added more restricted plans that included a smaller number of specific modes of treatment like acupuncture. Blue Cross has begun a test project ("AlternaPath") of coverage for naturopathy, homeopathy, and acupuncture that can be purchased alone or combined with a Blue Cross policy for conventional care. A company spokesperson called the response of consumers "overwhelming," and in mid-1997, California Blue Shield began to heavily promote its Lifepath preferred alternative provider plan in newspaper and radio ads.

It is already becoming clear that managed care companies are most interested in those modes of alternative therapy that can be described as procedures, like acupuncture, as opposed to systems, like Oriental or Ayurvedic medicine. Managed care accepts alternative medicine in the same way it accepts conventional care: as something that can be delivered in standardized units and evaluated with traditional outcome measures. Thus far, alternative medicine's ability to help managed care firms hold onto clients and add new ones seems to have been more important than its claims of reducing health care costs. William Sullivan, the CEO of Oxford Health Plans, commented, "The cynics say we're offering this because it's less expensive and that's simply not true. We're offering it because our membership told us this is what they wanted." He called the decision "a no brainer." The key issue for alternative medicine in its quest for integration into the medical mainstream is the degree to which it will lose its distinctive qualities, and itself be gobbled up as it assimilates. Will alternative medicine shape the mainstream, or will the mainstream recast the alternative through the force of assimilation to the norms of managed care and financial incentives?

The willingness of the government to accommodate alternative practitioners via licensure and other legislative means has also been frequently premised on the hope that the government's cost burden will decrease. As early as 1980, in his forward to *The Complete Guide to Holistic Medicine: Health for the Whole Person,* Senator Edward Kennedy promoted a more "holistic" approach to care. He noted that "we need to make changes in the kind of health care we provide to Americans as well as in its distribution and cost." In 1995, when Democratic Representative Jim Moran urged alternative medicine advocates to "inspire" their legislators to increase funds for OAM, he argued that "conventional medical treatments have become very expensive. . . . Alternative therapies . . . are an inherently more cost-effective approach to health and illness." Peter DeFazio, the Oregon Democrat who is the primary sponsor of the Access to Medical Treatment Act, which would facilitate the inclusion of most forms of non-FDA approved treatments in conventional medical settings, partly justifies the act in financial terms. He stated, "As we confront escalating medical costs and struggle to contain Medicare and Medicaid spending, alternative medicine becomes increasingly integral to the solution. . . . [It is] affordable, less invasive, and effective . . . especially in the areas of long term and chronic illness."

The executive branch of the government, largely via OAM, has become increasingly aware of the cost saving potential of integrating alternative techniques into conventional care. The Executive Summary of OAM's initial report to its parent National Institutes of Health stressed the goal of cost containment in its conclusion and recommendations. Wayne Jonas, OAM's current director, has established a section of the office on "professional and international liaison," with cost containment as a major focus, to coordinate work with third-party payers and licensing groups. The overwhelming concern at all levels of government is now with the cost of health care, as opposed to its efficacy or its ability to bring solace to the lives of the afflicted. Therefore, it should come as no surprise that alternative care is viewed in terms of cost. OAM's emphasis on alternative medicine as a cost-saving device appears to validate the early concerns that OAM might hasten the co-optation of alternative approaches by the larger system of care.

From Care to Commodity

The economics of alternative medicine in the United States are changing rapidly. As the absolute amount of money spent on alternative therapies and providers grows, the field is marked by consolidation and the emergence of a smaller number of much larger suppliers. Giant corporations, many in the communications industry, have become involved in the marketing of alternative therapies and approaches. Huge managed care plans are increasingly open to some forms of alternative care. The government is much more willing than ever to disseminate information about alternative therapies and sponsor research whose goal is not to debunk it, but to justify the inclusion of alternative approaches in the medical mainstream. The growing absolute and relative economic value of alternative medicine brings with it a growing legitimacy in the eyes of the society. This enhanced legitimacy then furthers its economic growth.

As alternative care is drawn into the mainstream of American life, economic forces become more and more decisive in determining what happens to it. The needs of all the major institutional players—managed care plans and insurance companies, large corporations, all levels of government, and the mass media—push toward a convergence of the alternative with the conventional.

In many respects, the situation is similar to the history of hospice care for the terminally ill. Hospices were developed in Great Britain with the aim of improving the quality of life for terminally ill patients. Their aim was to get patients out of traditional hospitals and into a free-standing environment where their special physical and psychological needs could be best met. Those who created the model and implemented it gave little, if any, consideration to its financial impact. But shortly after the idea was "imported" to the United States it became clear that the substitution of hospice care in place of inpatient care in a hospital would often be highly cost-effective. This recognition facilitated the rapid growth of hospices in managed care settings. But, over time, issues of reimbursement have come to redefine what constitutes hospice care in the United States. Today hospice typically consists of in-home care where services and equipment (hospital beds, etc.) are provided for a length of time that is determined by third party payers. Despite the growing acceptance of hospice care for the last six months of life by patients and providers, the length of time patients use the program has dropped sharply, from thirty-six to twenty-nine days between 1993 and 1995. Some programs offer excellent care, and the shift to home care, as opposed to institutional care, may benefit many patients. Still, the very nature of hospice has been altered by its immersion in the economic matrix of managed care. A similar process seems, to some degree, to be occurring as alternative therapy becomes a part of the larger managed care environment.

To date, chiropractic provides the clearest example of this process. Only twenty years ago the AMA was still calling chiropractic a "pseudomedical cult" and telling its members to boycott all contact with chiropractors. Over the past two decades chiropractic has been highly successful at integrating into the overall system of health care in this country. Today, many states require that comprehensive health care plans include coverage for chiropractic, and all major insurers and HMOs have lists of "preferred" chiropractors whose fees they reimburse. These developments occurred after a long history marked by both growing client demand for chiropractic services and legal challenges to exclusion, mounted by chiropractors. However, chiropractic under managed care is restricted to treatment for a few very specific conditions, and for a limited number of visits. Many chiropractors have been willing to abandon chiropractic's claims to be a system for treating the full range of illnesses in order to gain mainstream acceptance and the ability to practice in mainstream settings. Although a number of individuals, both within and outside of the chiropractic community, had long called for just such a limited role for chiropractic as an "allied health profession," it was the economic incentives and disincentives of managed care that brought it to fruition.

The emerging economic affinities between managed care organizations, chiropractors, and big business are increasingly apparent. In early 1996, the giant media conglomerate, Time Warner, began shipping over one million copies of a line of medical self-help videos to stores. The half-hour videos, which retail for $19.95, were produced by Patient Education Media, a firm jointly owned by a Time Warner subsidiary whose medical director is C. Everett Koop, the former Surgeon General. Cigna Healthcare, a large managed care firm, contracted to buy at least fifty thousand copies of various videos for use by its physicians and clients. According to Dr. W. Allen Schaffer, Cigna's senior vice president, the tapes are to be used with patients who have been diagnosed with a problem in order to make them aware of less costly options for treatment that their physicians might not normally discuss. The tape on back pain specifically discusses chiropractic as an option, as opposed to surgery. Currently, AT&T, IBM, and Microsoft all are developing interactive on-line health services, each of which includes a similar orientation toward chiropractic.

The economic benefits to firms like Time Warner don't come solely from mass marketing information on chiropractic or other alternative therapies. Users of Andrew Weil's website on the Internet, through Time Warner's Pathfinder personal computer network, will find ads for IBM, American Express, Barnes and Noble, and many other firms, along with omnipresent links to other Time Warner products: *People Magazine, Fortune, Money,* and others. Affluent consumers who want more information about their health are likely to want more information about how to manage their money, and many other topics. Such people are a target market for bookstores, computer companies, and many other businesses. Perhaps these firms hope that the confidence and respect the visitors to the website have for Dr. Weil will rub off on their products or services. Conversely, someone who initially seeks investment counsel by clicking onto the *Money Magazine* or *Fortune* site will find the link to Weil facing them.

In the broadest sense, information about alternative therapy has become a commodity. It generates profit, not only for those who produce and transmit it, but for those who associate themselves with it and for those who may indirectly gain financially through its use. To some significant degree, alternative medicine's ability to serve the economic needs of this diverse group is based in the fact that it relies heavily on direct contact and participation by the patient. Access to care is relatively unmediated by professional gatekeepers. Alternative providers market information about their services directly to prospective clients. The strength of large communication conglomerates lies in their ability to profit by directly mass marketing information. The managed care companies see potential cost savings when information on topics such as how to treat back pain or have a good diet can bypass the middlemen (physicians).

The mass media have played a crucial role in legitimizing alternative medicine. The generally favorable coverage of alternative medicine in *Time, Newsweek,* and many other publications offers the consistent message that alternative therapies are being widely used by educated, middle-class people, and that an informed, intelligent consumerism should prevail in assessing them. The implication, if not the explicit message, is: This is something our readers, or viewers should know about, and should consider using themselves.

The evolution of this perspective can be seen in the work of Jane Brody, the well-known and highly-regarded health writer with the *New York Times*. In the 1970s, Brody's columns and articles were generally skeptical about alternative medicine. But by 1996 her views had changed. One of her weekly "Personal Health" columns was captioned "Alternative medicine has its place in treatment and prevention. But be careful. Conventional doctors do not have all the answers." She described how her own experience seeking relief for an arthritic knee condition led her to use Alexander therapy and to try capsules available in a health food store, which she discovered contained the same substances "the veterinarian had prescribed for our arthritic dog." A few months later she wrote a follow-up column that said her knee had improved about 30 percent and that she was back to playing tennis and ice skating with less pain and no swelling in her knee. She noted that "I am only an anecdote of one, not a study that proves anything." A year later she added, "I continue to play singles tennis two to four times a week and skate four or five times a week, and I have added a daily three and a half mile brisk walk to my activities. Despite recent x-rays showing advanced arthritis in one knee and moderately advanced arthritis in the other, my knees do not swell anymore, and are no longer stiff after prolonged sitting." She also noted that as the drugs in question could not be patented, the drug companies had no incentive to ever conduct the needed research.

The *New York Times* reports on the widespread use of St. John's wort to treat chronic depression offer a telling example of how the mainstream media frequently treat information about alternative medicine. The *Times* has given this particular subject a good deal of attention. Its news articles have been straightforward and rather critical of the widespread use of this herbal remedy. On September 9, 1997, the *Times* devoted almost an entire page to the acceptance of the herb in Germany, where it outsells Prozac by four to one, and the

British Medical Journal's favorable review of twenty-eight different clinical trials. Still, the tone of the piece was skeptical, stressing the reservations that American physicians and drug companies had about St. John's wort. The sense of the article was summed up by the large boldface statement set off in the middle of the page: "Studies have yet to prove herb's effect on depression." But the very next day, Jane Brody's "Personal Health" column in the *Times* took a different tack. While voicing caution ("Keep in mind that the FDA does not approve the preparations of St. John's wort on the shelves of health food stores. . . ."), the article specified the doses of the herb that should be used ("look for brands containing 300 milligrams of the raw herb, standardized to contain 0.3 percent hypericin . . . take one capsule a day, less if you are older than 65"), and recommends a book and an 800 number for more information. Anyone reading the latter piece would come away feeling that the *Times* supported the use of the herb.

The September 1996 cover story in *Life Magazine*, "The Healing Revolution," even more explicitly legitimizes a convergence between alternative and conventional care. The photo on the cover shows a woman being cared for by a doctor using both a stethoscope and a sprig of herbs. The text reads "Surgery or acupuncture? Antibiotics or herbs? BOTH ARE BETTER. More and more M.D.'s are mixing Ancient Medicine and New Science to treat everything from the common cold to heart disease."

The economic affinities between alternative therapies, managed care, and big business are somewhat ironic. The inclusive character of many alternative approaches to healing, their emphasis on mind-body interventions, and their integration of spirituality and high-level functioning all create an "expanded" understanding of what qualifies as illness. The personal histories of most conventional physicians who have become oriented toward alternative medicine is marked by some sort of experience with their own illnesses, or spiritual growth that has convinced them that the traditional biomedical model of illness is too limited. Yet managed care and the corporations that pay for managed care through employee benefits have tended to favor a much more restricted understanding of what is "truly" an illness. How are these seemingly incompatible images of health care able to converge? The answer appears to be that the convergence is simultaneously taking place on two levels. Some alternative techniques are being integrated into managed care, largely on the basis of hoped for cost savings and their ability to serve as marketing tools. At the same time, a much broader set of alternative approaches are being promoted as legitimate but outside of conventional practice. The mass media make them accessible, for a price, to interested individuals, along with information on how to use, evaluate, and integrate them with conventional care.

Alternative medicine advocates usually assume that the validity and therapeutic utility of their practices will hasten some sort of convergence with, if not triumph over, conventional medicine. The reality is that the integration into conventional care that has occurred reflects the growing dominance of corporate life over all medicine. Alternative medicine is being judged according to the same standards as conventional medical techniques: for its ability to hold down costs and produce economic surplus. At the same time alternative approaches are thriving, in part because they, and information about them, have become consumer products that lend themselves to the most advanced forms of marketing. The commodification of alternative medicine has become the dominant theme in alternative medicine's relationship with managed care and the mass communications industry, as well as in the growth of its own institutions. The changes are buyer driven, as opposed to being driven by the professionals who produce the care.

8 The Future of Alternative Medicine

Alternative medicine plays a significant and growing role in American society. However, predictions about the future of alternative medicine frequently take one of two forms. Some advocates describe the future in glowing terms. They speak of a "medicine of great possibilities" that can effectively reduce the growing tide of chronic illness, significantly increase life expectancy, bring about dramatic cures, and even lead humankind to a higher, more fulfilled state. In reaching each of these lofty goals, alternative therapies will leave the world of conventional care far behind. Others see a very different future for alternative medicine. They predict the piecemeal assimilation of particular techniques into managed care settings and other large corporate providers on the basis of their ability to produce measurable, cost-effective outcomes in symptoms and client satisfaction. Some see this assimilation as a desirable outcome while others depict alternative medicine as shoring up the existing system of care as it becomes "a medicine of diminishing expectations." In this interpretation, patients are increasingly limited in their access to physicians and the technological wonders of modern medicine while they are told to "take responsibility for their own health." To what degree is each of these views realistic?

Assimilation and Cooptation

The case for alternative medicine's piecemeal integration into the medical mainstream under the near total control of conventional physicians and health care organizations is a powerful one. While "scientific medicine" may present itself as an exclusive club, with the most restrictive qualifications for membership, the historic reality is somewhat different. The boundaries between mainstream and alternative care have always been permeable, and conventional physicians have been willing to include just about any technique that seemed effective. Systems of care and types of healers that challenge the mainstream have the opportunity to become part of the dominant profession if they give up their claims to being unique. Osteopathy was once considered alternative. Today it is thriving (the number of osteopathic medical schools has grown from five to nineteen in the last thirty years) and fully integrated into the mainstream. But osteopathy's distinctive identity and therapies (a disdain for drugs and a reliance on muscular manipulation) have been nearly obliterated. More commonly, alternative approaches are incorporated under the domain of conventional providers, and their practitioners are offered limited rights as "allied" health care professionals. Although they have not necessarily acknowledged it, specialties like rehabilitative and physical medicine have long incorporated elements from massage and even chiropractic. Conventional physicians sometimes argue that there is no cohesive alternative point of view in order to justify the selective appropriation of particular alternative techniques into the mainstream, under their own control.

Perhaps the greatest force promoting the integration of alternative and mainstream therapies is the growing crescendo of consumer demand. For the most part, consumers are not interested in validating a particular model of medicine. They only seek to get well, alleviate their symptoms, or stay as healthy as they can. "Does it work?"—not "Is it mainstream or alternative?"—is their concern. Merrijoy Kelner and Beverly Wellman studied three hundred Canadian patients who used physicians, chiropractors, acupuncturists, naturopaths, and Reiki practitioners. They concluded that "Patients chose specific kinds of practitioners for particular problems, and some use a mixture of practitioners to treat a specific complaint. . . . The choice is multidimensional and cannot solely be explained by either disenchantment with medicine or by an 'alternative ideology.'"

Almost every study concurs: People who seek care from alternative providers also seek care from mainstream caregivers. As alternative care has become more widespread, combining mainstream and alternative modalities to deal with chronic illness has become the norm. Well over 90 percent of those suffering from conditions like arthritis use at least some alternative therapy. Some recent studies have found that over half of the patients visiting a primary care physician are simultaneously using alternative therapy for their problem. About half of these dual users do not disclose this fact to their physician. In the case of severe illnesses, the situation is similar. People with AIDS and their organizations inevitably favor a "multiple choice" strategy, as do those suffering from cancer and many other serious conditions. In reality, a rational consumerism and a critical skepticism about medicine can coexist with a traditional passive dependence on a conventional physician.

As I described in several of the earlier chapters, the assimilation of alternative approaches into conventional medicine is already well underway. Even the American Medical Association, the standard bearer for conservative forces within the profession, has shifted its views toward a more open stance. As late as the mid 1970s, the AMA's position was that "The fakes, the frauds, and the quackeries need to be identified, exposed, and, if possible, eradicated. This is not an easy task. The public is all too easily entranced with food fadism and pseudo-scientific diets. Legislators have been all too willing to incorporate chiropractic benefits into federal and state health care programs.

Uncontrolled acupuncture has been legalized in at least one jurisdiction." In those years the AMA's Committee on Quackery kept watch over all AMA publications to ensure they were keeping up the campaign against quackery. Through the mid 1970s, about forty critical reports per year on chiropractic appeared in *American Medical News,* the official newspaper of the AMA. But by 1995, the AMA's House of Delegates had substituted "alternative medicine" for the term "quackery" and passed a resolution that "our American Medical Association encourage its members to become better informed regarding the practices and techniques of alternative or complementary medicine."

This recent openness is reflected in the newer editions of the *AMA's Readers Guide to Alternative Health Methods,* as well as in the reviews of books on alternative medicine that appear in its publications, including *JAMA.* Typical is a 1995 review of *Choices in Healing: Integrating the Best Conventional and Complementary Approaches to Cancer,* authored by a political scientist ("I hear some physicians grumbling . . . Oh . . . Oh," the reviewer writes). The *JAMA* review calls the book the "best available single source" for information of use to the activist cancer patient. The review even concludes by chiding the author for not including a discussion of shark cartilage as a treatment for cancer and states, "The fascinating question is how many of these approaches will someday be embraced by contemporary, skeptical clinicians."

In late 1997, the *JAMA* editors and senior staff ranked alternative medicine as one of the three (out of eighty-six) most important subjects for the journal to address in the coming year. It had ranked sixty-eighth the year before. *JAMA*'s physician readers ranked it as seventh most important. One result of this newfound interest was that in November of 1998 the AMA made alternative medicine the sole focus of that month's JAMA, as well as the major theme in nine of its other journals. In all, about 80 research articles appeared. About half reported positive results from rigorously controlled clinical studies of alternative approaches to such problems as carpel tunnel syndrome (yoga), prostate enlargement (herbs), inflammatory bowel syndrome (herbs), and breech pregnancies (moxibustion—the burning of herbs near a specific point on the body, in this case, the big toe).

It has become commonplace to find articles in medical journals that stress the importance of clinicians understanding and accepting the "folk" beliefs of their clients. This often means an acceptance of the use of alternative therapies by the physician. One piece in *JAMA* advised allowing folk healers to deal with the "underlying causes" of illness, while physicians restrict themselves to treating symptoms. A similar view was recently espoused by an article in *The Annals of Internal Medicine,* which advised that a doctor "shutting the door" on a patient's desire for any less than scientific treatment is "the worst course of action." The article offers a detailed, week-by-week plan for doctors to use when their patients are also using alternative therapies, as well as a list of resources to help physicians find competent alternative therapists. The author concludes, "No patient should feel that their medical journey is to be taken alone or according to some stealth trajectory, invisible to their conventional providers. . . . The delivery of medical care, like the experience of illness, is best viewed as a journey shared."

Increasingly, conventional physicians appear to be following this advice. A majority of primary care physicians already are willing to refer their patients for therapies such as relaxation, biofeedback, hypnosis, and acupuncture, and one study of primary care M.D.'s found 80 percent believed that meditation or prayer had at least palliative power. Among contemporary medical specialties, family practice has become the most open to the basic premises of alternative care regarding prevention, the social basis of health, and the need for new strategies to deal with chronic illness. The inclusion of alternative material in the curricula of medical schools and residencies has been spearheaded by family practitioners and other primary care specialties. A similar situation has been documented in Britain.

As medical education has become more oriented toward primary health care, it too has been more willing to include material on alternative medicine. For example, at the Harvard Medical School the third- and fourth-year classes are now centered on the doctor-patient relationship. An instructor at the school noted that if he were to speak honestly, he could only detect "minor differences" between the premises of what was being taught and the alternative belief in "vitalism." The integration of alternative approaches into residency training for physicians is much less developed. But Andrew Weil's residency program at the University of Arizona is attempting to serve as a model for just such training for primary care physicians.

If primary care physicians are relatively open to alternative medicine, nurses and nurse practitioners are even more enthusiastic in embracing it. Nursing's longstanding emphasis on caring and the healing process, as opposed to curing, is itself based upon an implicit critique of conventional medicine. Over the past several years nursing has sought to differentiate itself from medicine and carve out a more independent base for autonomous clinical practice. This quest has been largely successful. Nurses now practice at least some form of primary care free of immediate supervision by doctors in forty-nine of the fifty states. In this context nurses have frequently seen alternative beliefs as an important foundation for their own professional efforts.

A growing openness on the part of many politicians, and governmental regulatory agencies, has enhanced mainstream medicine's receptivity toward alternative approaches. At the national level, the Office of Alternative Medicine plays a growing role in legitimizing specific alternative therapies, as well as alternative medicine as a whole. OAM has been especially effective in mobilizing the highly prestigious National Institutes of Health (NIH) to convene so-called "consensus conferences" on specific therapies such as relaxation techniques and acupuncture. The favorable reports from such conferences have received a great deal of publicity and have spurred local regulatory groups, HMOs, medical schools, and others to include these techniques among their activities. For example, the report on acupuncture, issued in November of 1997, called for its integration into standard medical practice to deal with nausea, chronic pain, and potentially many other problems. Insurers, managed care plans, Medicaid, and Medicare all explicitly urged the coverage of acupuncture. As described in Chapter 7, the forces of corporate medicine and managed care are usually receptive to the amalgamation of alternative techniques. They tend to view them as low-cost opportunities to build their markets, and possibly help their clients.

The mass media, which pay an increasing amount of attention to health and health care, embrace these efforts to assimilate alternative techniques. A 1997 *Los Angeles Times* list of what everyone should keep in their medicine cabinet, which took up almost the entire front page of that paper's weekly "Health Section," typifies the extent that the media accepts the integration of alternative and conventional care. The first six items listed under the subheading "What the Docs Say You Oughta Have" were echinacea for treatment of cold/flu; valerian to induce sleep; melatonin to help restore the body's clock; licorice root to ease coughing and sore throat; chamomile to alleviate digestive troubles; and feverfew to ease symptoms of migraine headaches, nausea and vomiting. Thermometer, ice pack, ace bandage, and CPR instructions followed about ten items later. The explosive growth of the Internet and other interactive information services promises to foster the integration of alternative and conventional approaches to an even greater degree.

Although most alternative practitioners and advocates see this process of assimilation as a good thing, some remain more reserved, and some are even hostile. They view the process not as integration, but as cooptation, which threatens to destroy what is unique about alternative care. They fear that integration into mainstream medicine's current environment of specialization, institutional consolidation, corporate control, and managed care will rip alternative techniques from the core beliefs upon which they are built. The time, caring, and effort necessary to reflect the values of holism, personal responsibility, and transcendence are simply not available or "reimbursable" in most conventional medical settings. When placed in this context, the power and meaning of alternative medicine can be lost. The alternative techniques are turned into commodities and doled out in the same way as conventional care. Still, given the forces of consumer demand—combined with the pressures from managed care, government, and the media—the "mainstreaming" of alternative medicine appears to be a certainty.

One need only look again to the mass media to find many examples of the sort of dilution and trivialization that advocates of alternative medicine fear. A typical case appears in *For Women First,* a magazine available at newsstands and supermarket checkout lines. The September 1995 issue featured an article entitled "Fast Results! Discover the Healing Power of AYURVEDA" on its cover along with articles on "The Best Hairstyles for Your Face" and "12 Things Thin Women Do Differently." The eight-page story on Ayurveda began with a twenty-four-item quiz to determine the reader's basic Ayurvedic type (vata, pitta, or kapha). On the basis of the quiz, the article made recommendations for stress reduction and for changing the reader's diet, skin care, activity level, and sexual response in order to "fine tune those out of balance problems that keep you from achieving perfect weight, beauty, and overall health." Although articles like this one may help acquaint some people with alternative medicine, the superficiality of the material, along with the grandiose claims, may do more to trivialize it as a form of narcissism.

Given the immense pressures driving toward integration, assimilation, and cooptation, it is not hard to see why most observers conclude that alternative medicine has a weak future as an independent institutional entity. While many alternative therapies and practitioners may move from being on the "fringe" of medicine to being an accepted complement to the mainstream, they will lose their own autonomy in the face of a more powerful set of assimilationist forces. The overwhelming range and power of these forces make it difficult to envision alternative medicine developing as a full-blown institutional presence. The ideological cohesiveness of alternative medicine, as expressed through its core beliefs, is not matched by its institutional reality. The limited independence of alternative medicine's organizations and institutions is likely to diminish even further in the future.

An Identity Movement

With its diffuse and permeable organizational boundaries, and vague or ephemeral qualities, what is alternative medicine? Some call it a social movement. For these observers, its movement status is based upon the consistency, coherence, and cogency of its "slogans," "model of health and illness," or "ideology." It is a movement based upon what Gusfield called "consciousness of kind." It is "a collective experience . . . [wherein] people . . . see themselves as having a common history . . . sharing symbols, legends . . . [and] attitudes towards events, both past and present."

Alternative medicine offers the possibility of reinterpreting a problem, or imagining a way of reframing a personal problem. In this sense it has the potential to be similar to feminism. Over the past several decades feminism, or "the women's movement," has had an immense impact upon countless individuals as well as on the society at large. The work of feminists has affected many aspects of women's daily lives including how they relate to physicians and do their jobs. Many women would consider feminism to have been a major influence on their own identities. Yet, relatively few women have belonged to a feminist organization or participated in formal movement activities. Feminism is an identity grafted on to other identities: mother, spouse, worker. It provided a "master frame" in which the inferior position of women could be transformed from an inevitability to an injustice. In the same manner, alternative medicine offers a "master frame" in which the misfortune of illness can be converted to an opportunity that can be addressed through action. In both cases the identity offered by the movement requires action on the part of the individual.

Renee Anspach has called this process the "decloseting" of deviance, while Kurt Back refers to the ability of an identity movement to "unfreeze" a situation. As in the case of other identity movements, alternative medicine uses its ideology, or core beliefs, to call forth a personal transformation on the part of its adherents. The power of so many specific alternative approaches comes in their ability to offer a detailed "map" to the road of personal transformation. Similar to many religious movements like evangelical Christianity, Eastern religious groups, and "new age" movements, alternative medicine offers the opportunity to confront personal issues and take action outside of traditional institutions through self-sufficiency and looking inward to one's self, family, and close friends. All of these movements stress the body-mind-spirit connection and individual transcendence as sources of healing.

Taken together, these movements have reinvigorated a set of beliefs that, despite their rich legacy, had fallen out of favor with society. Each emphasizes the role of nature, personal responsibility, the influence of mind and spirit on the body, and the ultimate meaning of health. The renewed vigor and appeal of these groups speaks, in part, to the immense spiritual hunger in the nation on the part of those who are ill, or of those who seek to improve their well being. This is a hunger that mainstream institutions, both medical and religious, appear ill equipped to satisfy. In simple terms, those who are sick, and those who want to be healthier, want what alternative medicine has to offer. They seek a sense of meaning about their condition, confidence that they can transcend to a better level of well-being, a sense of control over their destiny, a connection with forces outside of themselves, and a more equal and fulfilling relationship with those upon whom they rely for help.

Of course, like all these movements, alternative medicine runs the risk of becoming an ad hoc, superficial accumulation of ideas from various approaches to healing, religious traditions, and humanistic psychology, not to mention shamanism and transcendentalism. To many critics this conglomeration lends itself to replacing logic and scientific standards of evidence with a superficial, naive, "feel good" adoration of the self. Still, alternative medicine's existence as a vibrant, ongoing social movement around which people recreate their identities at times of great need is as much an undisputed reality as the assimilationist tendencies that limit its organizational presence.

Perhaps most important in assessing the future impact of alternative medicine as an identity-altering movement in American life is the fact that the underlying grievances to which it responds are becoming more pronounced. The organization and cost of health care, the neglect of prevention or mind-body dualism in medicine, and the lack of continuity and genuine caring among conventional providers are each increasingly seen as problems by both clients and policymakers. While the specialization of physicians, the corporate dominance of medicine, and the restrictions of managed care continue to grow rapidly, they have, if anything, heightened the criticism that the media, politicians, and the public voice towards medicine. In recent national surveys, more than half the respondents say that managed care has lowered the quality of care for those who are ill, and that their plans are more interested in saving money than in providing the necessary care.

The combination of pressures from managed care, high tech medicine, and the perceived risks of chronic illness will ensure that the educated populace will distance itself even more from conventional medicine over the coming years. There are two reasons for this. Ironically, the first factor is the very success of medical science and technology. High tech medicine can recreate our physical bodies through cosmetic and plastic surgery, the use of artificial organs, and transplants. Genetic medicine can "engineer" individuals outside of any living organism. All of these developments promise to widen the gulf between how medical scientists understand who we are and our own understanding of ourselves. Such medical "progress" has the effect of separating one's sense of self from one's perception of his/her body. In this environment, an alternative medicine that challenges these developments by integrating body and mind, and cherishes the sanctity of the whole person, becomes even more appealing.

The rising tide of chronic illness and disability is another factor that will heighten the appeal of alternative approaches. The number of Americans who suffer from such conditions is immense and growing. Today about half of the adult population suffers from at least one chronic illness. As the population ages, this proportion will increase rapidly. As knowledge about these conditions increases, both the medical and lay communities become more aware of their precursors. These "risk factors" determine the likelihood that an individual will be afflicted and, sometimes, determine the disease severity as well. Many important risk factors are at least partially modifiable via behavioral and attitudinal changes by the individual. Thus, more and more of the nation's adults have come to define themselves as "at risk" for some specific disease or diseases. This self-defined "at risk" population is highly motivated to initiate change. Yet, conventional medicine either downplays the importance of some risk factors, and or is not especially helpful in fostering and maintaining the necessary changes. This is especially the case for the mushrooming array of genetic and psychological risk factors. Here the risk is embodied within the individual and suggests that people have to change *who* they are, not only *what* they do. The executive editor of the

New England Journal of Medicine recently wrote an article for the public entitled "Overdosing on Health Risks . . . The best medical advice: Relax." Her position was, "Science has hardly begun to touch the big mysteries about diet and other habits. We simply do not know what is risky and what isn't, and what we do know is often distorted or misinterpreted." This is the attitude that drives many people toward, and not away from, alternative medicine. Yet, regardless of these views, medical research on the precursors of chronic illness has created a massive amount of new questions about diet, exercise, stress, and many other topics that conventional medicine is unable to address. The "pre-victimhood" of chronic illness has become an important part of middle-class, middle-age identity and a prime motivator of exposure to alternative medicine.

Thus, we see a bifurcation of alternative medicine. On the level of organization and institutions, both mainstream and alternative care are becoming integrated with alternative medicine in a subservient role and losing its independence. At the same time alternative medicine as a transformational identity is becoming more prominent throughout American life. This bifurcation of alternative medicine will be abetted by other developments as well. It is highly likely that research will continue to reinforce the contextual premises of alternative medicine's core beliefs that go beyond specific therapeutic techniques. For example, a 1997 report from the Society for Neuroscience meeting described how exercise can actually undermine health benefits if people don't "really want" to do it. It seems that forced exercise suppresses the immune system, while voluntary exercise enhances immune functioning. While the research was done on rats, the researchers presented their findings as probably applicable to humans and specifically stated "that the stress engendered by forced exercise programs for post heart attack patients may undermine the benefits of the exercise." In other words, it is the orientation of the individual toward the action, as opposed to the action in itself, that is either beneficial or harmful. While conventional medicine has little use for such a finding, it fits well within the core beliefs of alternative medicine, especially the view that individuals should be highly active, involved, and participatory in their own care.

Equally important to the continued prominence of alternative medicine is the way that the research finding described above became known. The research, on laboratory rats, was reported at a fairly obscure academic meeting. Yet the news media picked it up, distributed it to thousands of outlets, and described it on the Internet. This is an example of how the media crystallizes and shapes the public discourse. The researcher's statements about how the study might apply to humans came not from publications for a professional audience, but from media interviews. Science writers and editors have become "brokers," framing and sharpening a critical distancing from conventional medical perspectives. This process shows no sign of abating. If anything the role of the media is rapidly growing, and their thirst for stories that support the basic premises of alternative medicine (individual responsibility, the interpenetration of body-mind-spirit, prevention, and the transcendent attainment of "wellness") appears insatiable.

Today, those who are ill, and those who are well but consider themselves at risk for becoming ill, want to play a more active role in their own health and healing. The identity offered by alternative medicine provides a way to transcend the misfortune of illness and the day-to-day drudgery of maintaining good health. Illness, symptoms, and the deprivations of taking good care of yourself are converted into opportunities for improved self-esteem, personal growth, and even joy. Although it can be parodied and trivialized, often with some justification, the public's hunger for this perspective is quite genuine. As an identity movement, alternative medicine is driven by massive demand. The true contribution of alternative medicine is its ability to turn pathology into opportunity.

Notes

Chapter 1: The Emergence of Alternative Medicine

PAGES

2   **Cover stories:** *Life Magazine* Colt (1996), *Newsweek* Cowley (1996), *Time* Langone (1996), Wallis (1996).

3–4   **Cousins's quotation:** Cousins (1976:1459).

4–5   **Surveys on use of alternative therapies:** Eisenberg et al. (1998), Landmark Healthcare (1998), Astin (1998).

5   **Use of chiropractic:** Carey et al. (1995), Shekelle (1994).

5–6   **Use of alternative medicine by terminally ill:** Yates et al. (1993); **Overall use:** Cassileth and Brown (1988).

6   **Sales of natural foods:** Brooks (1996); **Sales of medicinal herbs:** *Los Angeles Times* (1995:D1).

6–7   **HMOs contracting for spiritual healing:** Hilts (1995).

7   **Survey of HMO executives:** John Templeton Foundation (1997); **NIH review on AIDS research:** Altman (1996); **Homeopathy in Britain:** Kleinjen et al. (1991).

9   **Moss books:** Moss (1993, 1996).

Chapter 2: Victims of Medicine

13   **The medicalization of life:** Illich (1976), Zola (1978), Conrad (1992).

14   **The alternative views of health that derive from Christian Science and Seventh Day Adventism:** Poloma (1991), Numbers (1976).

15   **The human being as an indivisible unit of mind and body:** Maslow (1987).

16   **Quotation on the placebo effect's implications for medicine:** Price (1984).

16–8   **Reviews of research on the power of the placebo effect:** Frank (1991), Price (1984).

18–9   **The impact of bereavement on mortality rates of those who survive:** Lynch (1977), Martikainen and Valkonen (1996).

PAGES
19   **Loneliness and isolation lead to poor health among primates:** Sapolsky (1990); **Hostile, cynical and hopeless feelings linked to atherosclerosis:** Everson et al. (1997); **Job characteristics relating to health:** Alfredsson et al. (1982), Kobasa (1982), Marmot (1994).

21   **Range of spiritually oriented self-help groups in the United States:** Wuthnow (1997); **Public opinion polls about belief in "alternative realities":** Froheck (1992), *Los Angeles Times* (1995); **Mystically oriented sites on the World Wide Web:** Pinkerton (1996).

21–2   **Survey of physicians on spirituality in their practice:** John Templeton Foundation (1996).

22   **Quotation on Asclepius:** Dubos (1959:114).

23   **The limited role of clinical medicine in reducing mortality:** McKinlay and McKinlay (1977), Evans and Stoddard (1990), and McKeown (1979); **Impact of social status, working conditions, and physical environment on health:** Antonovsky (1979), Berkman (1995), Schnall et al. (1990); **Calls for a "public health paradigm":** Evans and Stoddard (1990), Sobel (1995).

24–5   **Growth in health care spending:** Levit, Lazenby, and Sivarajan (1996), Pear (1998).

25   **Census Bureau report on health insurance coverage:** U.S. Bureau of the Census (1996); **U.S. health care expenditures on chronic conditions and Medicare:** Hoffman, Rice, and Sung (1996), Health Care Financing Administration (1995); **Aging population increasing Medicare costs:** Schneider and Guralnik (1990).

25–6   **Inefficiency of the U.S. health care system:** Woolhandler and Himmelstein (1997).

26   **Impact of medical spending on health status of population:** Wolfe (1986), Evans and Stoddard (1990); **Rise of managed care:** Jensen et al. (1997), Drake (1997), Health Systems Review (1996).

27   **1997 Harris Poll on managed care:** Kilborn (1997).

28   **1994 *Chicago Tribune* report about falsified research:** Associated Press (1994).

29   **Quotations about recommendations on mammography:** Kolata (1997).

30   **Percentage of U.S. women having hysterectomies:** Payer (1988); **Political boundaries influencing utilization of medi-**

PAGES

cal procedures: Wennberg (1984); **Clinical decision-making is a matter of social norms and values:** Askham (1982), Frieman (1985).

31   Physical exams not useful for screening asymptomatic illness: Oboler and Laforce (1989); **Harm of "PSA" screening exam:** Krahn et al. (1994); **Coincidence of back pain and disc abnormalities:** Jensen et al. (1994); **Radiologists disagree on mammograms:** Ellmore et al. (1994); **Faulty elderly medical records:** Beers, Munekata, and Storrie (1990); **Patients injured by medical treatment:** Brennan et al. (1991); **Physicians' misuse of pharmaceuticals:** Morse (1986); **Adverse drug reactions kill:** Grady (1998).

32   Contradictory opinions on pain control: Bionica (1991), Roan (1996); **1978 report on proportion of medical procedures that work:** Office of Technology Assessment (1978); **Little improvement in medical efficacy since 1978:** Banta and Thatcher (1990).

33–4   Consumerism and medical care: Roter et al. (1997), Emanuel and Emanuel (1992).

34   Beta carotene: Cimons (1996); **Spinal manipulation:** Rosenthal (1991); **Herbal remedies:** Monmaney (1996); **Diet and relaxation:** Brody (1996a,b); **Melatonin:** Cowley (1995); **Declassification of homosexuality as an "illness":** Bayer (1981).

35   Quotation from *The New Our Bodies, Ourselves:* Boston Women's Health Collective (1984:556).

37   **"Paradigm shift":** Kuhn (1970).

37–8   Kuhn on the applicability of his ideas beyond physics: van Gelder (1966).

38   Quotations describing alternative medicine as a unique paradigm: Chopra (1993:5), Alster (1989:8), Pelletier (1979: 23–24).

Chapter 3: The Core of Alternative Medicine: Age-Old Wisdom Made New

41   Irrationality and foolishness as essence of alternative medicine: Relman (1981), Fitzgerald (1983).

43   Quotation on lack of uniformity in holism: Vanderpool (1984:773); **Classification of common elements of alternative medicine:** Gordon (1990), Buckman and Sabbagh (1995), O'Connor (1995), Alster (1989), Lowenberg (1989).

PAGES

45   **Quotation on each person requiring a different approach:**
            Gordon (1980:16–17); **Quotation on homeopathy consider-
            ing the patients' "wholeness":** Coulter (1980:397, emphasis
            in original).

46   **Quotation on modern medicine considering symptoms
            only:** Johnston (1991:38–41).

46–7   **Chopra's quotation on Ayurveda:** Chopra (1989:142).

47   **Traditional Chinese Medicine:** Mann (1974), Beau (1972),
            Kaptchuk (1992); **Naturopathy:** Weil (1988), Murray and Piz-
            zorno (1989).

48   **Unhappy people suffer from more disorders:** Selye (1956),
            Antonovsky (1979), Schnall et al. (1990), Haynes, Feinleib, and
            Kannel (1980), Linkins and Comstock (1990), Everson et al.
            (1997); **PNI:** Borysenko (1988), Kiecolt-Glaser and Glaser
            (1988).

48–9   **People can control the process of PNI:** Kabat-Zinn (1990),
            Achterberg (1985), Benson (1993).

49   *JAMA* **study on sadness and blood supply:** Mittleman and
            McClure (1997); **The power of the mind over the body op-
            erates indirectly:** Weil (1988:235).

50   **Eliminating warts:** Weil (1988); **TCM, Ayurveda, and yoga
            all connect mind, body, and spirit:** Beinfield and Korngold
            (1995:45), Chopra (1989, 1991, 1993), Frawley (1990), Vish-
            nudevananda (1980), Iyengar (1987); **Popularity of Transcen-
            dental Meditation:** Chalmers et al. (1989).

50–1   **Impact of meditation on physiological processes:** Alexander,
            Schneider, and Staggers (1996), Knight (1995), MacLean et al.
            (1994).

51   **Meditation and spiritual enlightenment:** Shapiro and Walsh
            (1984), Borysenko (1988), Kabat-Zinn (1990); **Biofeedback
            and guided imagery treat a range of disorders:** Kamiya and
            Kamiya (1980), Gruber et al. (1993), Rees (1993), Ilacqua
            (1994), Zachariae et al. (1994), Stevenson (1995); **Guided im-
            agery fights cancer and AIDS:** Hay (1994); **Guided imagery
            derives from TCM and Ayurveda:** Naparstek (1994:52).

51–2   **Physical manipulation techniques employ mind-body inter-
            action:** Frager (1980).

52   **Nonspecific mind-body interactions:** Rolf (1977), Alexander
            (1969), Barlow (1991); **Specific mind-body interactions:**
            Feldenkrais (1992), Heller and Henkin (1991); **Hellerwork:**
            Lowen (1975), Lowen and Lowen (1977).

Jahnke (1990); **Dean Ornish's dietary regimen for cardio-vascular problems:** Ornish (1990); **Quarter of prescription drugs derived from plants:** Farnsworth et al. (1985).

64 **Cousins on his relationship with his doctor:** Cousins (1976: 1463).

65 **The importance of the clients' motivations and expectations:** Kamiya and Kamiya (1980), Achterberg (1985), Weil (1988); **Dossey on "healing words":** (Dossey 1993).

66 **Remen on imagery:** Remen (1992); **:Quotations from Dossey on love and healing:** Dossey (1993:109, 117).

67 **Accounts of personal transformations among alternative healers:** Montgomery (1996); **Quotations on personal experiences of American Holistic Medical Association members:** Goldstein et al. (1985), Goldstein et al. (1987).

67–8 **Frank on healing:** Frank (1975, 1991).

70 **Alternative medicine as heretical challenge to orthodoxy:** Wolpe (1990).

Chapter 4: Medicine and the Spirit

75 **Ayurvedic and the Vedic tradition:** Lad (1995), Chopra (1989); **TCM, acupuncture, and Taoism:** Bresler (1980), Beinfield and Korngold (1991); **Quotation on Innate Intelligence in chiropractic:** Martin (1994:212); **Spiritual nature of chiropractic and homeopathy:** Palmer (1917), Fuller (1989: 25); **Herbal remedies:** Hoffman (1996), Tierra (1992); **Meditation and hypnosis:** Shapiro and Walsh (1984), Cardena (1994).

76 **Prayer as healing:** Dossey (1993).

77–8 **Survey on American's belief in god and quotation on religion's influence on politics:** Pew Research Center (1996).

78 **1996 poll of scientists:** Larson and Witham (1997).

78–9 **TIME/CNN poll on prayer and illness:** Wallis (1996:62).

79 **Gallup Poll on near-death experiences:** Ring (1980); **Surveys on American religious belief/National Opinion Research Center survey:** Briggs (1984), General Social Survey (1997).

80 **A third of Americans report being in contact with a spiritual force:** Levin (1993).

81 **Review of over 250 studies showing effect of religion on**

PAGES

health: Levin and Schiller (1987); **Kibbutz study:** Kark et al. (1996).

82   **Kuopio Ischemic Health Disease Risk Factor Study:** Rasanen et al. (1996); **Study on death and religious service attendance:** Stawbridge et al. (1997); **Faith and open heart surgery:** Oxman, Freeman, and Manheimer (1995).

82–3   **Religious practice, immune function, and recovery:** Koenig et al. (1997), Azhar et al. (1994).

83   **Religious beliefs and good health:** Levin (1994); **Mormon practice and lung cancer:** Gardner and Lyon (1982a,b).

84   **Levin on spirituality and health:** Levin (1993, 1994, 1996a,b).

85   **Dossey's work on spirituality and health:** Dossey (1982, 1989, 1993); **Benor's work on people using thought to manipulate physical characteristics:** Benor (1990).

85–6   **Dossey on "new physics" and healing:** Dossey (1993:xv–8, 41–42, 205).

87–8   *New England Journal of Medicine* **"sounding board" essay:** Glymour and Stalker (1983:961, 963).

88   *JAMA* **conflict with Chopra:** Sharma, Triguna, and Chopra (1991).

88–9   *JAMA* **editor's response:** Skolnick (1991).

89   **Spirituality and health providers:** Montgomery (1996), Lowenberg (1989).

90   **Study of American Holistic Medical Association:** Goldstein et al. (1987, 1988).

90–1   **Omission of fasting's religious origins:** Burton Goldberg Group (1993:224).

91   **Quotations on nineteenth century healers and animal magnetism:** Fuller (1989:9, 48).

92   **Quotation on Eastern mystical traditions:** Fuller (1989:94).

93–4   **The Relaxation Response:** Benson (1993); **Quotations from Timeless Healing:** Benson (1996b:203, 183, 177, 196, 305, 299).

94   **Therapeutic Touch:** Krieger (1988), McCrae (1992).

94–5   **Weil's 8 Week Plan:** Weil (1997a).

95   **Weil on spirituality and religion:** Weil [1997a:24–25 (emphasis added), 28], Weil (1997b, 1988:42).

97   **Dossey's quotations on prayer:** Dossey (1993:8, 84); **on magic:** (ibid., 155–156, italics in original); **Pelletier on new paradigm:** Pelletier (1979:187, 217).

PAGES
97–8   **Ornish quotation on old ideas:** quoted in Horrigan (1995a:92).

98   *Lancet* **study on homeopathy for allergies:** Reilly et al. (1994); **Reilly quotation on being a shaman:** Horrigan (1995b:70, 73).

99   **Holton's critique:** Holton (1992:106); **Chopra quotation on fiction:** in Biema (1996).

99–100   **The Gates of Eden:** Gross and Levitt (1994).

100   **Alternative medicine as "nonsecular" spirituality:** Bradshaw (1996:415, 416).

102   **Dossey quotation on importance of meaning in health:** Dossey (1995a:10).

102–3   **Survey of family practice physicians:** John Templeton Foundation (1996).

103   **Benson on teaching prayer:** Hilts (1995); **Physicians should include spiritual dimension:** Dacher (1995).

103–4   **Friedman quotation on doctors asking patients about their belief system:** Hilts (1995).

104–5   **Dossey's "guide" to prayer:** (1993, ch. 5).

105   **Dossey on hidden agenda:** Dossey (1993:99).

107   **1996 Supreme Court case:** Carter (1996).

108   **Screening instruments to determine who will benefit from spiritual interventions:** Daaleman and Nease (1994); **Quotation on monistic religions:** Robbins and Anthony (1979:77).

109   **Chopra quotation on spirituality:** Leland and Power (1997).

Chapter 5: Is There *Really* an Alternative Medicine?

111   **Gordon on a "holistic paradigm":** Gordon (1980); **Quotation from *Alternative Medicine: The Definitive Guide:*** Burton Goldberg Group (1993:14–15); **Quotation from *Alternative Healing: The Complete A–Z Guide:*** Kastner and Burroughs (1996).

112–3   **Chopra quotations on Ayurveda:** Chopra (1989:5, 13, 237).

113   **Chopra quotation on bliss:** Chopra (1993:329); **Chopra quotation on chi:** Chopra (1993:262); **Chopra quotation on a new paradigm:** Chopra (1993:21).

114   **Quotation on mission from *Alternative Therapies:*** (1995:4); **Dossey quotation on a lingua franca:** Dossey (1995b:7).

116   **Goals of the AHMA:** American Holistic Medical Association

PAGES

(1997), **Goals of the AHNA:** American Holistic Nursing Association (1997).

116–7   **Goals of PATH:** Professional Association of Traditional Healers (1996).

117   **Symposium on alternative medicine:** International Spa and Fitness Association (1995).

119   **Quotation on mission from _Alternative Therapies:_** Alternative Therapies (1995:4).

119–120   **Quotation on the California Institute of Integral Studies:** California Institute of Integral Studies (n.d.:24).

120   **Quotations on the Arizona Program in Integrative Medicine:** Weil (1997b).

120–1   **Micozzi on The Complete Wellness institutions:** Micozzi (1996).

121   **Salmon and Berliner on the holistic health movement:** Salmon and Berliner (1980).

122   **Sale quotations on fluidity of practice boundaries:** Sale (1995:13, 50).

123   **Hufford quotation on the language of health:** Hufford (1995:56); **OAM's budget increase:** Office of Alternative Medicine (1997:3).

124   **Quotation from AMA House of Delegates:** American Medical Association (1973:34).

125   **Quotation from AMA consumer guidebook:** Zwicky et al. (1993); _Time_ **magazine quotation on alternative medicine:** Langone (1996:42); **Relman quotation:** MacFarquhar (1997:31).

125–6   **Surveys show doctors don't understand why alternative treatments are effective:** Ernst et al. (1995), Berman et al. (1995).

126   **Harkin quotations on alternative therapies:** Harkin (1995:71).

127   **NIH funds university research centers:** Office of Alternative Medicine (1998); **Medical schools with courses on alternative medicine:** Wetzel, Eisenberg, and Kaptchuk (1998); **Success of alternative clinics:** Thomson (1996).

128   **Quotation on Oxford coverage of alternative medicine:** _New York Times_ (1996); **American Society of Clinical Oncology:** Reuters (1997a); **Quotation on American Cancer Society:** American Association for Holistic Health (1997); **Quota-**

tion on the American Medical Association resolution: Colt (1996).

129   *JAMA* article on therapeutic touch: Rosa et al. (1998); O'Connor on alternative therapies and AIDS: O'Connor (1995).

130   Quotation on AIDS panel recommendations: Altmann (1996).

130-1   *New York Times Magazine* article on cancer: Lerner (1994).

131   Holistic Health Directory: *New Age Journal* (1995-96); Example of locally produced directory: Laughing Dragon Publications (1995).

132   Casper on the Alternative Health and Healing Forum: AHH Pulse (1997); AMRTA: Alchemical Medicine Research and Teaching Association (1997); Quackwatch site: Quackwatch (1998).

132-3   Webwatch: *Yoga Journal* (1997:16).

133   Quotation from editorial in *Homeopathy Today*: *Homeopathy Today* (1994:2).

134   Quotation on nature of a collective identity: Johnston et al. (1994:16-17).

135   Gusfield on social movements and holistic health: Gusfield (1994:65, 69); A "critical distance" from conventional scientific medicine: Williams and Calnan (1996).

138   Quotation from the NHF: National Health Foundation (1995); Quotation from *Alternative Healing: The Complete A–Z Guide to More than 150 Alternative Therapies*: Kastner and Borroughs (1966).

139   Weber on the overconsumption of food: Turner (1982); Physical exercise, piety, and civility: Struna (1981); American health crusaders: Whorton (1982), Schwartz (1986), Levenstein (1988).

139-140   Quotations from the Omega Institute catalogue: Omega Institute (1997:84).

140   Quotations from Whole Life Expo: Whole Life Expo (1996:27); Chopra quotation on unlimited wealth: Chopra (1994:55).

141   Quotation on new social movement: Melucci (1994).

Chapter 6: The Politics of Alternative Medicine: Personal and Practical

143   **Simonton quotation:** Simonton, Mathews-Simonton, and Creighton (1978:115).

144   **Hay quotation on 100% responsibility for our experiences:** Hay (1994:5); **Choosing one's parents:** Hay (1994:10); **Quotations on choice:** Jampolsky (1979:156), Shealy and Myss (1993:123).

144–5   **Szasz quotation on illness politics:** Szasz (1975:166).

146   **Anti-science worldview:** Holton (1992:120–121); **Laetrile:** Cancer Control Society (1996a,b).

146–7   **Right-wing political agenda of Laetrile advocates:** Markle et al. (1978).

147–8   **John Birch Society website on Laetrile:** John Birch Society (1997).

148   **National Health Federation quotation on mission:** National Health Federation (n.d.).

148–9   **Health Freedom News quotations:** National Health Federation (1995:10).

149–150   *Perceptions* **quotations:** Betah Foundation (1996:2, 30).

150   **Jampolsky on God's will:** Jampolsky (1989:156); **Eastern religions and "liberal" political views:** Robbins and Anthony (1979).

151   **Freire quotation:** Freire (1970:36).

152   **Lowenberg quotations:** Lowenberg (1989:171, 179).

153   **Research Center for Alternative Medicine mission:** Research Center for Alternative Medicine (1997); **Nineteenth century feminism and alternative medicine:** Goldsmith (1998); **Quotation from** *The New Our Bodies, Ourselves:* Boston Women's Health Collective (1984:xiii).

158   **CBS News poll:** Berke (1997); **Weil website quotation on marijuana legalization:** Weil (1997b); **Weil on innate desire for altered states of consciousness:** Weil and Rosen (1993); **"Green" medicine:** Ullman (1986).

159   **Quotations on alternative medicine's goals:** Burton Goldberg Group (1993:17–18).

161   **Quotation on the AHMA:** American Holistic Medical Association (1997).

162   **Quotation on the AHNA:** American Holistic Nursing Association (1997).

PAGES

163–4   **Starr on medicine's autonomy:** Starr (1982).

164   **Common pattern among health providers of allowing future restrictions in exchange for current autonomy and high income:** Freidson (1970), Berlant (1975), Starr (1982).

164–5   **Quotation on owning massage:** Muscat (1995).

165   *Consumer Reports* **on homeopathy:** *Consumer Reports* (1994:203, 206).

166–7   **Fetzer Institute findings:** Sale (1995:50–51).

167–8   *Newsweek* **article:** Seligmann and Cowley (1995:68).

168–9   *New York Times* **articles:** Kolata (1996a).

169   **FDA decisions on ephedra:** Bass (1997); *New York Times* **op-ed piece:** Friedman (1996).

170–1   **Burzynski:** Smith (1992), Burzynski Research Institute (1997).

171–2   **Range of state-wide regulations of massage:** Beck (1996).

173   **Moran quotation:** Moran (1995).

174   **Harkin quotation:** Harkin (1995); **DeFazio quotation:** DeFazio (1996).

175   **Dossey quotation on Newt, Bill, and Hillary:** Chowka (1996:157).

176   **Quotation on purpose of OAM:** Trachtman (1994).

177   **Quotation on special offices' lack of control over research:** *Journal of NIH Research* (1996); **Jacobs quotation on NIH's limited view:** Trachtman (1994:115).

178   *New York Times* **quotation on the gulf between NIH and OAM:** Angier (1994); **Jacobs's resignation:** Marshall (1994).

179   **Insider bias at OAM:** Motz (1994); **Jonas's guiding principle:** Office of Alternative Medicine (1995:4).

180   **Hildenbrand quotation:** Villaire (1995); *New York Times* **articles:** Kolata (1996a–c); *New York Times* **op-ed piece:** Park and Goodenough (1996).

180–1   **Jacobs and Jonas responses:** Jacobs (1996), Jonas (1996).

181   **Porter quotation:** Porter (1995).

182   **AIDS panel recommendations:** Altman (1996); **Behavioral medicine conference conclusions:** Chilton (1996); **JAMA summary paper on relaxation techniques:** NIH Technology Assessment Panel (1996); **Making acupuncture reimbursable under Medicare:** Office of Alternative Medicine (1994).

183   **Metropolitan King County council unanimous approval of naturopathic clinic:** Egan (1996), Bland (1995).

Chapter 7: Alternative Medicine, Mainstream Markets

185   **Study on amount spent on alternative providers:** Eisenberg et al. (1998).

186   **Entrepreneurial aspects of alternative practices:** Young (1961), Gevitz (1988), Armstrong and Armstrong (1991); **ELF bracelet:** Bioelectric Research (n.d.).

186–7   **Magnet mattress:** Body Magnetics (n.d.).

187   **Homeopathic aphrodisiacs:** RB Distribution (1996); **Trampolines:** Walker (1995); **Aloe vera:** R Pure Aloe International (n.d.); **Blue green algae:** Cell Tech (1992); **Neon lights:** Enlightened Concepts (n.d.); **Journey portraits:** Fairrington (1996); **Hawaiian noni fruit distributors:** Weil (1997b).

188   **200-page nationwide directory:** *New Age Journal* (1995–96).

189   **Hoxsey therapy, hydrazine sulfate, Issel's Whole Body therapy, Kelley's Nutritional metabolic therapy, shark cartilage, Livingston therapy, Revici Therapy:** Duarte (1993), Gerson (1990), Hoxey (1956), Livingston-Wheeler (1984), Walters (1993).

189–190 **Quotation from the Gerson clinic:** Gerson (1990).

192   **Chopra book sales post–Oprah Winfrey show:** Biema (1996).

194   **Medicinal herb sales:** Oldham (1995); **Organic produce and bottled water sales:** Burros (1996).

195   **The market for homeopathic remedies:** Gorman (1992).

195–6   **Percent of natural food sales in supermarkets:** *Natural Foods Merchandiser* quoted in Brooks (1996).

197   *Newsweek* **cover story on melatonin:** Cowley (1995); **Ten herbs account for over half of all sales:** Herb Research Foundation, cited in Brooks (1996).

197–8   **Wisconsin ginseng:** Iritani (1998).

198   **Isolating ginseng's active ingredient:** Brooks (1996); **Merging of organic food superstores:** Murphy (1996); **Chains control 20 percent of natural foods market:** Brooks (1996).

199   **Median income of** *Prevention* **readers:** Rodale Press (1996).

200   *JAMA* **report on chronic conditions:** Hoffman, Rice, and Sung (1996); **Little "choice and voice":** Mechanic and Rochefort (1996).

201   **Doctor-patient interaction unsatisfying:** Roter et al. (1997).

204   **Jacobs quotation:** Jacobs, Jennifer (1995:48); **Quotation on qigong:** Burton Goldberg Group (1993:431).

204–5   **Quotation from** *Natural Health:* Thomson (1996:102).

PAGES

205   **Lippin quotation:** Lippin (1996:51); *JAMA* **editorial:** Callan (1979).

206   **Quotation in** *Western Journal of Medicine* **on cooptation:** Carlson (1979:470).

207   **St. John's wort trial:** Linde et al. (1996); *New England Journal of Medicine* **article:** Carey et al. (1995); *American Journal of Hypertension* **article:** Shapiro et al. (1997).

208   **Benson quotation on money in the bank:** Hilts (1995); **Quotation on "Spirituality and Healing" conference tapes:** Harvard Medical School (1996).

209   **Ornish quotation on cost savings:** Ornish (1995:88); **Estimated savings for Mutual of Omaha:** Turner (1995); **Survey on alternative therapy requests at HMOs:** Landmark Healthcare (1996); **HMOs offer acupuncture:** Olmos (1997).

210   **California Blue Shield's Lifepath:** Office of Alternative Medicine (1997); **Sullivan quotations:** ABC News (1997).

211   **Kennedy quotation:** Kennedy (1980:ix); **Moran quotation:** Moran (1995:79); **DeFazio quotation:** DeFazio (1996:94); **OAM's initial report:** Office of Alternative Medicine (1992: xxvi, xxvii); **Section of OAM on "professional and international liaison":** Jonas (1996).

212   **Early concern about cooptation of OAM:** Motz (1994).

214   **Time Warner tape on back pain:** Freudenheim (1996).

216   **Quotation from Brody column caption:** Brody (1996c); **Quotation from follow-up column:** Brody (1997a); **Brody quotation on tennis-playing:** Brody (1998).

217   *New York Times* **quotation on St. John's wort:** Andrews (1997), Brody (1997b); *Life Magazine* **cover story:** Colt (1996).

Chapter 8: The Future of Alternative Medicine

221   **Quotation on Canadian study:** Kelner and Wellman (1997:203); **Arthritis sufferers' use of alternative therapy:** Kronenfeld and Wasner (1982); **Dual users don't tell physicians:** Spencer and Jonas (1997); **People with AIDS use multiple strategies:** O'Connor (1995).

221–2 **Quotation from AMA on uncontrolled acupuncture:** American Medical Association (1973:34); **Quotation from AMA resolution on being better informed about alternative medicine:** American Medical Association (1995:410); *Choices in*

Healing: Integrating the Best Conventional and Complementary Approaches to Cancer: Lerner (1994); **Quotation from** *JAMA* **review:** Merrill (1995); **How** *JAMA***'s readers ranked alternative medicine:** Fontanarosa and Lundberg (1997).

223   *JAMA* **piece on folk healers:** Pachter (1994); **Quotation from** *Annals of Internal Medicine* **on shared journey:** Eisenberg (1997); **Physicians willing to refer patients:** Blumberg et al. (1995); **Physician study on power of prayer:** John Templeton Foundation (1996); **Similarities in Britain:** Tovey (1997).

223–4 **Medical school teachings similar to vitalism:** Kaptchuk (1997:20).

224   **Nurses use alternative medicine as basis of autonomous practice:** Watson (1995).

225   *Los Angeles Times* **list for medicine cabinets:** Miller (1997).

226   *For Women First* **quiz on Ayurveda:** Noonan (1995:10); **Assimilation will weaken independence of alternative medicine:** Cant and Calnan (1991).

227   **Alternative medicine as a social movement:** Alster (1989), Lowenberg (1989), Mattson (1982), Sharma (1992); **Gusfield quotation:** Gusfield (1975:35).

227–8 **Master frame:** Turner (1992).

228   **The "decloseting" of deviance:** Anspach (1979); **Unfreezing:** Back (1987).

229   **Surveys on quality of managed care:** Kilborn (1997).

229–230 **High tech medicine confuses our understanding of ourselves:** Williams (1997).

230   **Percent of aging population suffering from chronic disease:** Hoffman, Rice, and Sung (1996).

230–1 **Article by the editor of the** *New England Journal of Medicine:* Angell (1997).

231   **Quotation on Society for Neuroscience report:** Reuters (1997b).

Bibliography

ABC News. 1997. Managed Alternatives. URL *http://www.abcnews. com/sections/nc . . . wnt0915_hmo.alternatives/index.html* (visited 10/20/97).

Achterberg, J. 1985. *Imagery in Healing: Shamanism and Modern Medicine.* Boston, MA: New Science Library/Shambala.

AHH Pulse. 1997. Alternative Health and Healing Homepage. URL *http://www.tile.net/lists/ahhpulse.html* (visited 12/1/97).

Alchemical Medicine and Teaching Association (AMRTA) 1997. Homepage. URL *http://amrta.org* (visited 4/15/97).

Alexander, C. N., et al. 1996. Trial of Stress Reduction for Hypertension in Older African-Americans. *Hypertension* 28: 228–237.

Alexander, F. M. 1969. *The Resurrection of the Body.* New York: Delta.

Alfredsson, L., R. Karasek, and T. Theorell. 1982. Myocardial Infarction Risk and Psychosocial Work Environment: An Analysis of the Male Swedish Working Force. *Social Science and Medicine* 16: 463–467.

Altman, L. K. 1996. Panel Offers Sharp Criticism of AIDS Research Programs. *New York Times* 14 March: A1.

Alster, K. B. 1989. *The Holistic Health Movement.* Tuscaloosa: The University of Alabama Press.

Alternative Therapies. 1995. 1 (1). Masthead: 4.

American Association for Holistic Health. 1997. Wellness for Life! *The Official Newsletter of the American Association for Holistic Health.* Spring issue.

American Holistic Medical Association (AHMA). 1997. Homepage. URL *http://www.ahma.org* (visited 04/15/97).

American Holistic Nursing Association (AHNA). 1997. Homepage. URL *http://www.ahna.org* (visited 4/15/97).

American Medical Association. 1973. *Proceeding of the House of Delegates.* New York.

American Medical Association. 1995. *Proceedings of the House of Delegates.* Chicago.

Andrews, E. C. 1997. In Germany, Humble Herb is a Rival to Prozac. *New York Times* 9 September: B1.

Angell, M. 1997. Overdosing on Health Risks. *New York Times Magazine* 4 May: 44–45.

Angier, N. 1994. U. S. Head of Alternative Medicine Quits. *New York Times* 1 August: A9.

Anspach, R. 1979. From Stigma to identity Politics. *Social Science and Medicine* 13A: 765–773.

Antonovsky, A. 1979. *Health, Stress, and Coping.* San Francisco: Jossey-Bass.

Armstrong, D., and E. Armstrong. 1991. *The Great American Medicine Show.* New York. Prentice-Hall.

Askham, J. 1982. Professionals' Criteria for Accepting People as Patients. *Social Science and Medicine* 16: 2083–2089.

Associated Press. 1994. 11 April. 16 May. AP Internet News. URL *http: //www.ap.org/* (visited 4/16/94).

Astin, J. A. 1998. Why People Use Alternative Medicine: Results of a National Study. *Journal of the American Medical Association* 279:1548–1553.

Azhar, M., et al. 1994. Religious Psychotherapy in Anxiety Disorder Patients. *Acta Psychiatria Scandinavica* 90: 1–3.

Bach, E., and Wheeler, F. J. 1979. *The Bach Flower Remedies.* New Caanan, CT: Keats.

Back, K. 1987. The Logic of Socially Innovative Movements. *Journal for the Theory of Social Behavior* 17: 161–180.

Banta, D., and S. Thatcher. 1990. The Case for Reassessment of Health Care Technology. *Journal of the American Medical Association* 264: 235–240.

Barlow, W. 1991. *The Alexander Technique.* New York: Alfred A. Knopf.

Bass, D. 1997. FDA Proposes Limits on Natural Stimulant. *New York Times* 15 June: E3.

Bayer R. 1981. *Homosexuality and American Psychiatry: The Politics of Diagnosis.* New York: Basic.

Beau, G. 1972. *Chinese Medicine.* New York: Avon Books.

Beck, R. L. 1996. An Overview of State Alternative Healing Practice Law. *Alternative Therapies* 2(1): 31–34.

Beers, M. H., M. Munekata, and M. Storrie. 1990. The Accuracy of Medication Histories in the Hospital Medical Records of Elderly Persons. *Journal of the American Geriatrics Society* 38: 1183–1187.

Beinfield, H., and E. Korngold. 1991. *Between Heaven and Earth: A Guide to Chinese Medicine.* New York: Ballantine Books.

Beinfield, H., and E. Korngold. 1995. Chinese Traditional Medicine: An Introductory Overview. *Alternative Therapies* 1 (1): 44–52.

Bellah, R., et al. 1996. *Habits of the Heart: Individualism and Commitment in American Life* (updated ed.). Berkeley, CA: University of California Press.

Benor, D. J. 1990. Survey of Spiritual Healing Research. *Complimentary Medical Research* 4: 9–33.

Benson, H. 1975. *The Relaxation Response.* New York: Avon.

Benson, H. 1996. *Timeless Healing: The Power and Biology of Belief.* New York: Scribner Books.

Berke, R. 1997. Suddenly the New Politics of Morality. *New York Times* 15 June: E3.

Berkman, L. 1995. The Role of Social Relations in Health Promotion. *Psychosomatic Medicine* 57: 245–254.

Berlant, J. 1975. *Profession and Monopoly.* Berkeley, CA: University of California Press.

Berman, B., et al. 1995. Physicians' Attitudes Toward Complementary or Alternative Medicine: A Regional Survey. *Journal of the American Board of Family Practice* 8: 361–366.

Betah Foundation. 1996. *Perceptions* 3 (March/April): 2, 30.

Biema, D. V. 1996. Of the Soul. *Time Magazine* 24 June: 65–67.

Bioelectric Research. n.d. The ELF Bracelet: Electromagnetic Revolutions. Silver Springs, NV: pamphlet.

Bionica, J. J. 1991. History of Pain Concepts and Pain Therapy. *Mt. Sinai Journal of Medicine* 58: 191–202.

Bland, J. S. 1995. Diet and Prostrate Problems. *Alternative Therapies* 1(4): 75–76.

Blumberg, D., et al. 1995. The Physician and Unconventional Medicine. *Alternative Therapies* 1(3): 31–35.

Body Magnetics. n.d. Magnetic Therapy Products. Suffield, CT: sales catalog.

Borysenko, J. 1988. *Minding the Body, Mending the Mind.* New York: Bantam.

Boston Women's Health Collective. 1984. *The New Our Bodies, Ourselves.* New York: Simon and Schuster.

Bradshaw, A. 1996. The Spiritual Dimension of Hospice: The Secularization of an Ideal. *Social Science and Medicine* 43: 409–419.

Brennan, T. A., et al. 1991. Incidence of Adverse Events and Neglect in Hospitalized Patients: Results of the Harvard Medical Practice Study I. *New England Journal of Medicine* 324: 370–376.

Bresler, D. E. 1980. Chinese Medicine and Holistic Health. Edited by A. C. Hastings, J. Fadiman, and J. S. Gordon. *Health for the Whole Person.* Boulder, CO: Westview Press.

Briggs, K. A. 1984. Religious Feeling Seen Strong in U.S. *New York Times* 9 December: 35.

Brody, J. 1996a. Relaxation Method May Aid Health. *New York Times* 7 August: B6.

Brody, J. 1996b. Strict Diet Rivals Drugs for Blood Pressure. *New York Times* 14 November: A14.

Brody, J. 1996c. Personal Health. *New York Times* 13 November: B7.

Brody, J. 1997a. Taking an Alternative Path to Search for Relief for Arthritic Knees. *New York Times* 15 January: B10.

Brody, J. 1997b. Personal Health. *New York Times* 10 September: B10.

Brody, J. 1998. The Arthritis is at Bay, Thank You. *New York Times* 13 January: B17.

Brooks, N. R. 1996. From Gooch to High Gloss: Change Signals Shift for Natural Foods Industry. *Los Angeles Times* 24 July: D1.

Brown, E. R. 1979. *Rockefeller Medicine Men*. Berkeley, CA: University of California Press.

Buckman, R., and K. Sabbagh. 1995. *Magic or Medicine?: An Investigation of Healing and Healers*. Toronto: Key Porter Books.

Burros, M. 1996. A New Goal Beyond Organic: Clean Food. *New York Times* 7 February: B1.

Burton Goldberg Group. 1993. *Alternative Medicine: The Definitive Guide*. Puyallup, WA: Future Medicine Publishing, Inc.

Burzynski Research Institute. 1997. Antineoplastons—FDA Declares War. URL *http://cancermed.com/antineo3.htm* (visited 3/5/97).

California Institute of Integral Studies. n.d. Catalog of course offerings.

Callan, J. 1979. Holistic Health or Holistic Hoax. *Journal of the American Medical Association* 241: 1156.

Cancer Control Society. 1996a. Tijuana, Mexico Clinics Tour Advertisement.

Cancer Control Society. 1996b. Symposium brochure.

Cant, S. L., and M. Calnan. 1991. On the Margins of the Medical Marketplace? An Exploratory Study of Alternative Practitioners' Perceptions. *Sociology of Health and Illness* 13: 39–57.

Cardena, E. 1994. Just Floating in the Sky: A Comparison of Hypnotic and Shamanistic Phenomena. *Yearbook of Cross-Cultural Medicine and Psychotherapy*. 85–98.

Carey, T. S., et al. 1995. Care-Seeking Among Individuals with Chronic Low-Back Pain. *Spine* 21: 312–317.

Carlson, R. J. 1979. Holism and Reductionism as Perspectives in Medicine and Patient Care. *Western Journal of Medicine* 131: 466–470.

Carter, S. L. 1996. The Power of Prayer, Denied. *New York Times* 31 January: A13.

Cassileth, B. R., and H. Brown. 1988. Unorthodox Cancer Medicine. *Ca—A Cancer Journal for Clinicians* 38: 176–186.

Cell Tech. 1992. Super Blue-Green Algae: The Key. Newsletter (December). Klamath Falls, OR.

Chalmers R. A., et al. 1989. *Scientific Research on Maharishi's Transcendental Meditation and TM-Sidhi Program, Volumes 2–4*. Vlodrop, The Netherlands: Maharishi Vedic University Press.

Chilton, M. 1996. Panel Recommends Integrating Behavioral and Relaxation Approaches into Medical Treatment of Chronic Pain, Insomnia. *Alternative Therapies* 2(1): 18–28.

Chopra, D. 1989. *Quantum Healing: Exploring the Frontiers of Mind-Body Medicine*. New York: Bantam Books.

Chopra, D. 1991. *Perfect Health*. New York: Harmony Books.

Chopra, D. 1993. *Ageless Body, Timeless Mind: The Quantum Alternative to Growing Old*. New York: Harmony Books.

Chopra, D. 1994. The Seven Spiritual Laws of Success. San Rafael, CA: Amber-Allen Publishing and New World Library.

Chowka, P. 1996. Prayer is Good Medicine. *Yoga Journal* July/August: 61–67, 156–158.

Cimons, M. 1996. Beta Carotene Won't Reduce Cancer Risk, Studies Show. *Los Angeles Times* 19 January: A1.

Colt, G. H. 1996. The Healing Revolution. *Life Magazine* September: 35–50.

Conrad, P. 1992. Medicalization and Social Control. *Annual Review of Sociology* 18: 209–232.

Consumer Reports. 1994. Homeopathy: Much Ado About Nothing? *Consumer Reports* March: 201–206.

Coplan-Griffiths, M. 1991. *Dynamic Chiropractic Today: The Complete and Authoritative Guide to This Major Therapy*. San Francisco, CA: Harper-Collins.

Coulter, H. L. 1980. Homeopathic Medicine. Edited by A. C. Hastings, J. Fadiman, and J. S. Gordon. *Health for the Whole Person*. Boulder, CO: Westview Press.

Cousins, N. 1976. Anatomy of an Illness: As Perceived by the Patient. *New England Journal of Medicine* 295: 1458–1463.

Cowley, G. 1995. Melatonin Mania. *Newsweek Magazine* 6 November: 60–63.

Cranton, E. 1990. *Bypassing Bypass*. Troutdale, VA: Hampton Roads.

Daaleman, T., and D. Nease. 1994. Patient Attitudes Regarding Physician Inquiry into Spiritual and Religious Issues. *Journal of Family Practice* 39: 564–568.

Dacher, E. S. 1995. Reinventing Primary Care. *Alternative Therapies* 1(5): 29–34.

DeFazio, P. 1996. Why Its Time for the Access to Medical Treatment Act. *Alternative Therapies* 2(1): 94.

Dosch, P. 1985. *Manual of Neural Therapy According to Huneke*. Heidelberg, Germany: Karl Haug Publishers.

Dossey, L. 1982. *Space, Time and Medicine*. Boston: New Science Library.

Dossey, L. 1989. *Recovering the Soul: A Scientific and Spiritual Search*. New York: Bantam.

Dossey, L. 1993. *Healing Words: The Power of Prayer and the Practice of Medicine*. San Francisco: HarperCollins.

Dossey, L. 1995a. What Does Illness Mean? *Alternative Therapies* 1(3): 6–10.

Dossey, L. 1995b. A Journal and a Journey. *Alternative Therapies* 1(1): 6–9.

Drake, D. 1997. Managed Care: A Product of Market Dynamics. *Journal of the American Medical Association* 277: 560–563.

Duarte, A. 1993. *Jaws for Life: The Story of Shark Cartilage*. Grass Valley, CA: Duarte Press.

Dubos, R. J. 1959. *The Mirage of Health*. London: Allen and Unwin.

Egan, T. 1996. Seattle Officials Seeking to Establish a Subsidized Natural Medicine Clinic. *New York Times* 3 January: A6.

Eisenberg, D. M. 1997. Advising Patients Who Use Alternative Medical Therapies. *Annals of Internal Medicine* 127: 61–69.

Eisenberg, D. M., et al. 1993. Unconventional Medicine in the United States: Prevalence, Costs, and Patterns of Use. *New England Journal of Medicine* 328: 246–252.

Eisenberg, D. M., et al. 1998. Trends in Alternative Medicine Use in the United States, 1990–1997: Results of a Follow-up National Survey. *Journal of the American Medical Association* 280:1569–1575.

Ellmore, J. G., et al. 1994. Variability in Radiologists' Interpretation of Mammograms. *New England Journal of Medicine* 331: 1493–1499.

Emanuel, E. J., and L. L. Emanuel. 1992. Four Models of the Patient Practitioner Relationship. *Journal of the American Medical Association* 267: 2221–2226.

Engle, G. L. 1977. The Need for a New Medical Model: A Challenge for Biomedicine. *Science* 196(4286): 129–135.

Enlightened Concepts, n.d. Advertising pamphlet. Beverly Hills, CA.

Ernst, E., et al. 1995. Complementary Medicine: What Physicians Think of It. *Archives of Internal Medicine* 155: 2405–2408.

Evans, R. W., and G. L. Stoddard. 1990. Producing Health, Consuming Health Care. *Social Science and Medicine* 31: 1347–1363.

Everson, S. A., et al. 1997. Hostility and Increased Risk of Mortality and Acute Myocardial Infarction: The Mediating Role of Behavioral Risk Factors. *American Journal of Epidemiology* 146: 142–152.

Fairrington, D. 1996. Heal Thyself. Journey Portraits. Advertising Flyer.

Farnsworth, N. R., et al. 1985. Medicinal Plants in Therapy. *Bulletin of the World Health Organization* 63: 965–981.

Feldenkrais, M. 1992. *The Potent Self: A Guide to Spontaneity.* San Francisco: Harper and Row.

Fitzgerald, F. T. 1983. Science and Scam: Alternative Thought Patterns in Alternative Health Care. *New England Journal of Medicine* 309: 1066–1067.

Fontanarosa, P., and G. Lundberg. 1997. Complementary, Alternative and Unconventional and Integrative Medicine. *Journal of the American Medical Association* 278: 2111–2112.

Frager, R. 1980. Touch: Working With the Body. Edited by A. C. Hastings, J. Fadiman, and J. S. Gordon. *Health for the Whole Person.* Boulder, CO: Westview Press.

Frank J. D. 1975. Mind-Body Relationships in Illness and Healing. *Preventive Medicine* 2: 46–59.

Frank, J. D. 1991. *Persuasion and Healing: A Comparative Study of Psychotherapy.* Baltimore, MD: Johns Hopkins University Press.

Frawley, D. 1990. *Ayurvedic Healing.* Salt Lake City: Morson Publishing.

Freidson, E. 1970. *Profession of Medicine.* New York: Dodd, Mead.

Freire, P. 1970. *Pedagogy of the Oppressed.* New York: Seabury Press.

Freudenheim, M. 1996. Time Warner Plans to Sell Medical Self-Help Videos. *New York Times* 22 February: C2.

Friedman, R. A. 1996. Natural Doesn't Mean Safe. *New York Times* 19 April: A17.

Frieman, M. P. 1985. The Rate of Adoption of New Procedures Among Physicians: The Impact of Specialty and Practice Characteristics. *Medical Care* 23: 939–945.

Froheck, F. M. 1992. *Healing Powers: Alternative Medicine, Spiritual Communities and the State.* Chicago: University of Chicago Press.

Fuller, R. C. 1989. *Alternative Medicine and American Religious Life.* New York: Oxford Press.

Gardner, J. W., and J. L. Lyon. 1982a. Cancer in Utah Mormon Men by Lay Priesthood Level. *American Journal of Epidemiology* 116: 243–257.

Gardner, J. W., and J. L. Lyon. 1982b. Cancer in Utah Mormon Women by Church Activity Level. *American Journal of Epidemiology* 116: 258–267.

General Social Survey. 1997. Data extracted from indices for 1983–1987 available at the University at Michigan Institute for Social Research. URL *http://www.icpsr.umich.edu/GSS/* (visited 11/5/97).

Gerson, M. 1990. *A Cancer Therapy: Results of Fifty Cases* (5th ed.). Bonita, CA: Gerson Institute.

Gevitz, N. 1988. *Other Healers: Unorthodox Healers in America*. Baltimore, MD: Johns Hopkins University Press.

Glymour, C., and D. Stalker. 1983. Engineers, Cranks, Physicians, Magicians. *New England Journal of Medicine* 308: 960–964.

Goldsmith, B. 1998. *Other Powers: The Age of Suffrage, Spiritualism, and the Scandalous*. New York: Knopf.

Goldstein, M. S. 1992. *The Health Movement: Promoting Fitness in America*. New York: Twayne/Macmillan.

Goldstein, M. S., et al. 1985. Holistic Doctors: Becoming a Nontraditional Medical Practitioner. *Urban Life* 14: 317–344.

Goldstein, M. S., et al. 1987. Holistic Physicians: Implications for the Study of the Medical Profession. *Journal of Health and Social Behavior* 28: 103–119.

Goldstein, M. S., et al. 1988. Holistic Physicians and Family Practitioners: Similarities, Differences, and Implications for Health Policy. *Social Science and Medicine* 26: 853–861.

Goodheart, G. 1989. *You'll Be Better: The Story of Applied Kinesiology*. Geneva, OH: AK Printing.

Gordon, J. S. 1980. The Paradigm of Holistic Medicine. Edited by A. C. Hastings, J. Fadiman, and J. S. Gordon. *Health for the Whole Person*. Boulder, CO: Westview Press.

Gorman, J. 1992. Take a Little Deadly Nightshade and You'll Feel Better. *New York Times Magazine* August 30: 23–28.

Grady, D. 1998. Reactions to Prescribed Drugs Kill Thousands Annually, Study Says. *New York Times* 15 April: A1.

Gross, P. R., and N. Levitt. 1994. *Higher Superstition: The Academic Left and its Quarrels with Science*. Baltimore, MD: Johns Hopkins University Press.

Gruber, B. L., et al. 1993. Immunological Responses of Breast Cancer Patients to Behavioral Interventions. *Biofeedback and Self Regulation* 18: 1–22.

Gusfield, J. R. 1975. *Community: A Critical Response*. New York: Harper and Row.

Gusfield, J. R. 1994. The Reflexivity of Social Movements. Pp. 58–78. *New Social Movements*. Edited by E. Larana, H. Johnston, and J. Gusfield. Philadelphia: Temple University Press.

Harkin, T. 1995. The Third Approach. *Alternative Therapies* 1(1): 71.

Harvard Medical School. 1996. Spirituality and Healing in Medicine: The Complete Conference in Video. Brochure and letter from S. Goldfinger, Faculty Dean of Continuing Education. Cambridge, MA: April 22.

Hay, L. 1994. *You Can Heal Your Life*. Santa Monica California: Hay House.

Haynes, S. G., M. Feinleib, and W. B. Kannel. 1980. The Relationship of Psychosocial Factors to Coronary Heart Disease in the Framingham Study, III: Eight Year Incidence of Coronary Heart Disease. *American Journal of Epidemiology* 111: 37–58.

Health Care Financing Administration. 1995. Medicare: A profile. Washington, D.C. *Health Care Financing Administration Chart* PS-11.

Health Systems Review. 1996. Charting the New Delivery Universe. *Health Systems Review* July/August: 28–37.

Heller, J., and Henkin, W. 1991. *Bodywise*. Berkeley, CA: Wingbow Press.

Hilts, P. J. 1995. Health Maintenance Organizations Are Turning to Spiritual Healing. *New York Times* 27 December: B10.

Hoffman, C., D. Rice, and H. Y. Sung. 1996. Persons with Chronic Conditions: Their Prevalence and Cost. *Journal of the American Medical Association* 276: 1473–1479.

Hoffman, D. 1996. *The Complete Illustrated Holistic Herbal*. Rockport, MA: Element Books.

Holton, G. 1992. How to Think About the Anti-Science Phenomenon. *Public Understanding of Science* 1: 103–128.

Homeopathy Today. 1994. Editorial. October: 2.

Horrigan, B. 1995a. Dean Ornish, M.D.: Healing the Heart, Reversing the Disease. *Alternative Therapies* 1(5): 84–92.

Horrigan, B. 1995b. David Reilly: Research, Homeopathy and Therapeutic Consultation. *Alternative Therapies* 1(4): 65–73.

Hoxey, H. 1956. *You Don't Have to Die*. New York: Milestone Books.

Hufford, D. J. 1995. Cultural and Social Perspectives on Alternative Medicine. *Alternative Therapies* 1(1): 53–60.

Ilacqua, G. E. 1994. Migraine Headaches: Coping Efficacy of Guided Imagery Training. *Headache* 34: 99–102.

Illich, I. C. 1976. *Medical Nemesis*. New York: Random House.

International Spa and Fitness Association. 1995. Advertising circular.

Iritani, E. 1998. Ginseng: Root for the Home Team. *Los Angeles Times* 12 March: A1.

Iyengar, B. K. S. 1987. *Light on Yoga*. New York: Schocken Books.

Jacobs, Jennifer. 1995. Homeopathy Should be Integrated Into Mainstream Medicine. *Alternative Therapies* 1(4): 48–53.

Jacobs, Joseph. 1995. Building Bridges Between Two Worlds: The NIH Office of Alternative Medicine. *Academic Medicine* 70: 40–41.

Jacobs, Joseph. 1996. Letter to editor. *New York Times* 9 January: A14.

Jaffe, D. T. 1988. *Healing From Within*. New York: Simon and Schuster.

Jahnke, R. 1990. *The Most Profound Medicine*. Santa Barbara, CA: Health Action Books.

Jampolsky, G. G. 1979. *Love is Letting Go of Fear.* Millbrae, CA: Celestial Arts.

Jampolsky, G. G. 1989. Pp. 156 *Healers on Healing.* Edited by R. Carlson and B. Shield. Los Angeles, CA: Tascher/Putnam.

Jensen, M. C., et al. 1994. Magnetic Resonance Imaging of the Lower Spine in People Without Back Pain. *New England Journal of Medicine* 331: 69–73.

John Birch Society. 1997. Homepage. URL *http://www.jbs.org* (visited 7/25/97).

John Templeton Foundation. 1996. Family Physicians' Survey. Radmor, PA.

John Templeton Foundation. 1997. Press Release. Survey Reveals HMO Executives overwhelmingly Recognize Role of Spirituality in Health Care. URL *http://www.templeton.org/sandh/course97/release3.htm* (visited 12/17/97).

Johnston, H., et al. 1994. Identities, Grievances, and New Social Movements. Pp. 3–35 in *New Social Movements.* Edited by E. Larana, H. Johnston, and J. Gusfield. Philadelphia: Temple University Press.

Johnston, L. 1991. *Everyday Miracles: Homeopathy in Action.* Van Nuys, CA: Christine Kent Agency.

Jonas, W. 1996. Letter to editor. *New York Times* 9 January: A14.

Journal of NIH Research. 1996. A Plethora of NIH Program Offices: Boon or Burden? 8: 25–27.

Kabat-Zinn, J. 1990. *Full Catastrophe Living.* New York: Dell.

Kamiya, J., and J. G. Kamiya, 1980. Biofeedback. In *Health for the Whole Person.* Edited by A. C. Hastings, J. Fadiman, and J. S. Gordon. Boulder, CO: Westview Press.

Kaptchuk, T. 1992. *The Web That Has No Weaver: Understanding Chinese Medicine.* New York: Congdon and Weed.

Kaptchuk, T. 1997. The Gap Between Conventional Medicine and Alternative Medicine. *Annual Report of European Commission on Unconventional Medicine.* Brussels: Commission of the European Communities. 20–22.

Kark, J. D., et al. 1996. Does Religious Observance Promote Health? Mortality in Secular vs. Religious Kibbutzim in Israel. *American Journal of Public Health* 86: 341–346.

Kaslof, L. J. 1988. *The Bach Remedies: A Self-Help Guide.* New Caanan, CT: Keats.

Kastner, M., and B. Burroughs. 1996. *Alternative Healing: The Complete A–Z Guide to More than 150 Alternative Therapies.* New York: Henry Holt and Company/Owl Books.

Kelner, M., and B. Wellman. 1997. Health Care and Consumers' Choice: Medical and Alternative Therapies. *Social Science and Medicine* 45: 203–212.

Kennedy, E. 1980. Forward in *Health for the Whole Person*. Edited by A. Hastings, J. Fadiman, and J. S. Gordon. Boulder, CO: Westview Press. ix–x.

Kiecolt-Glaser, J., and R. Glaser, 1988. Psychological Influences on Immunity: Implications for AIDS. *American Psychologist* 43: 892–898.

Kilborn, P. 1997. Dissatisfaction is Growing with Managed Care Plans; Quality of Services is Doubted, Survey Says. *New York Times* 28 September: 12.

Kleinjen, J., et al. 1991. Clinical Trials of Homeopathy. *British Medical Journal* 302: 316–323.

Knight, S. 1995. Use of Transcendental Meditation To Relieve Stress and Promote Health. *British Journal of Nursing* 4: 315–318.

Kobasa, S. C., S. R. Madi, and S. Kahn. 1982. Hardiness and Health: A Prospective Study. *Journal of Personality and Social Psychology* 42: 168–177.

Koenig, H. G., et al. 1997. Attendance at Religious Services, Interleukin-6, and Other Biological Indications of Immune Function in Older Adults. *International Journal of Psychiatry in Medicine* 27: 233–250.

Kolata, G. 1996a. On Fringes of Health Care, Untested Therapies Thrive. *New York Times* 17 June: A1.

Kolata, G. 1996b. In Quests Outside Mainstream, Medical Projects Rewrite Rules. *New York Times* 18 June: A1.

Kolata, G. 1996c. Doctor's Cancer "Cure" Attacked by FDA. *New York Times* 24 July: A1.

Kolata, G. 1997. Stand on Mammograms Greeted with Outrage. *New York Times* 28 January, C7.

Krahn, M. D., et al. 1994. Screening for Prostate Cancer: A Decision Analytic View. *Journal of the American Medical Association* 272: 773–780.

Krieger, D. 1988. *Living the Therapeutic Touch: Healing as Lifestyle*. Wheaton, IL: Quest Books.

Kronenfeld, J., and C. Wasner. 1982. The Use of Unorthodox Therapies and Marginal Practitioners. *Social Science and Medicine* 16: 1119–1125.

Kuhn, T. S. 1970. *The Structure of Scientific Revolutions* (2nd ed.). Chicago: The University of Chicago Press.

Lad, V. 1995. An Introduction to Ayurveda. *Alternative Therapies* 1(3): 57–63.

Landmark Healthcare. 1996. Health Maintenance Organizations and Alternative Medicine: A Closer Look. Report. Sacramento, CA.

Landmark Healthcare. 1998. The Landmark Report on Public Perceptions of Alternative Care. Report. Sacramento, CA.

Langone, J. 1996. Alternative Therapies: Challenging the Mainstream. *Time Magazine* Fall Special Issue: 40–43.

Larson, E. J., and L. Witham. 1997. Scientists Are Still Keeping the Faith. *Nature* 386: 435–436.

Laughing Dragon Publications. 1995. Directory of Alternative Health Care. East Sound, WA.

Leland, J., and C. Power. 1997. Deepak's Instant Karma. *Newsweek* 20 October: 52–60.

Lerner, M. 1994. *Choices in Healing: Integrating the Best Conventional and Complementary Approaches to Cancer.* Cambridge, MA: MIT Press.

Levenstein, H. 1988. *Revolution at the Table: The Transformation of the American Diet.* New York: Oxford University Press.

Levin, J. S. 1993. Age Differences in Mystical Experience. *The Gerontologist* 33: 507–513.

Levin, J. S. 1994. Religion and Health: Is There an Association, Is it Valid, Is It Causal? *Social Science and Medicine* 28: 1475–1482.

Levin, J. S. 1996a. How Religion Influences Morbidity and Health: Reflections on Matural History, Salutogenesis and Host Resistance. *Social Science and Medicine* 43: 849–864.

Levin, J. S. 1996b. How Prayer Heals: A Theoretical Model. *Alternative Therapies* 2(1): 66–73.

Levin, J. S., and P. L. Schiller. 1987. Is There a Religious Factor in Health? *Journal of Religion and Health* 26: 9–36.

Levit, K. R., H. C. Lazenby, and L. Sivarajan. 1996. Health Care Spending in 1994: The Slowest in Decades. *Health Affairs* 15: 130–144.

Lincoln, Y. S. 1992. Fourth Generation Evaluation, The Paradigm Revolution, and Health Promotion. *Canadian Journal of Public Health* 183 (Supplement 1): S6–S10.

Linde, K., et al. 1996. St. John's Wort for Depression: An Overview and Meta-analysis of Randomized Clinical Trials. *British Journal of Medicine* 33: 253–258.

Linkins, R. W., and G. W. Comstock. 1990. Depressed Mood and Development of Cancer. *American Journal of Epidemiology* 132: 962–972.

Lippin, R. 1996. Alternative Medicine in the Workplace. *Alternative Therapies* 2(1): 47–51.

Livingston-Wheeler, V. 1984. *The Conquest of Cancer.* San Diego, CA: Waterside Productions.

Loeser, J. D. 1994. The Prevention of Needless Pain. *Preventive Medicine* 23: 709.

Los Angeles Times. 1995. A Profitable Age. 4 August: D1.

Lowen, A. 1975. *Bioenergetics.* New York: Penguin Books.

Lowen, A., and L. Lowen. 1977. *The Way to Vibrant Health: A Manual of Bioenergetic Exercises.* New York: Harper.

Lowenberg, J. S. 1989. *Caring and Responsibility.* Philadelphia: University of Pennsylvania Press.

Lynch, J. J. 1977. *The Broken Heart: The Medical Consequences of Loneliness.* New York: Basic Books.

MacFarquhar, L. 1997. Andrew Weil, Shaman, M.D. *New York Times Magazine* 24 August: 28–31.

MacLean, C. R., et al. 1994. Altered Responses of Cortisol, GH, TSH, and Testosterone to Acute Stress after Four Months' Practice of Transcendental Meditation (TM). *Annals of the New York Academy of Sciences* 764: 381–384.

Mann, F. 1974. *The Treatment of Disease With Acupuncture.* Philadelphia: International Ideas.

Markle, G., et al. 1978. Notes from the Cancer Underground: Participation in the Laetrile Movement. *Social Science and Medicine* 12: 31–37.

Marmot, M. G. 1994. Social Differentials in Health Within and Between Populations. *Daedalus* 123: 197–215.

Marshall, E. 1994. The Politics of Alternative Medicine. *Science* 365: 2000–2002.

Martikainen, P., and T. Valkonen. 1996. Mortality After the Death of a Spouse: Rates and Causes of Death in a Large Finnish Cohort. *American Journal of Public Health* 86: 1087–1093.

Martin, S. C. 1994. The Only Truly Scientific Method of Healing. *Isis* 85: 207–227.

Maslow, A. 1987. *Motivation and Personality.* New York: Viking.

Mattson, P. H. 1982. *Holistic Health in Perspective.* Palo Alto, CA: Mayfield Publishing.

McCrae, J. 1992. *Therapeutic Touch: A Practical Guide.* New York: Knopf.

McKeown, T. 1979. *The Role of Medicine: Dream, Mirage or Nemesis?* Princeton, NJ: Princeton University Press.

McKinlay, J. B., and S. McKinlay. 1977. The Questionable Contribution of Medical Measures to the Decline of Mortality in the Twentieth Century. *Milbank Memorial Fund Quarterly* 55: 405–428.

Mechanic, D., and D. A. Rochefort. 1996. Comparative Medical Systems. *Annual Review of Sociology* 22: 239–270.

Melucci, A. 1994. A Strange Kind of Newness. What's "New" in New Social Movements? Pp. 101–130 in *New Social Movements.* Edited by E. Larana, H. Johnston, and J. Gusfield. Philadelphia: Temple University Press.

Merrill, J. M. 1995. Review of M. Lerner. Choices in Healing. *Journal of the American Medical Association* 273: 597.

Micozzi, M. (ed.) 1996. *Fundamentals of Complementary and Alternative Medicine.* Portland, OR: Churchill Livingston.

Miller, M. 1997. Will Your Medicine Cabinet Save Your Life? *Los Angeles Times* 15 September: S1.

Mittleman, M., and M. McClure. 1997. Mental Stress During Daily Life Triggers Myocardial Ischemia. *Journal of the American Medical Association* 277: 1558–1559.

Monmaney, T. 1996. Herb May Help Ease Depression, Studies Show. *Los Angeles Times* 2 August: A26.

Montgomery, C. L. 1996. The Care-Giving Relationship. *Alternative Therapies* 2(2): 52–57.

Moran, J. 1995. Making Alternative Therapies Everyone's Issue. *Alternative Therapies* 1 (4): 79.

Morse, L. M. 1986. Therapeutic Drug Use Review Reduces Incidence of Drug Related Illness. *Business and Health* 3: 58.

Moss, R. 1993. *Cancer Therapy: The Independent Consumer's Guide to Non-Toxic Treatment and Prevention.* Brooklyn, NY: Equinox Press.

Moss, R. 1996. *The Cancer Industry: The Classic Exposé on the Cancer Establishment.* Brooklyn, NY: Equinox Press.

Motz, J. 1994. Healing Hopes: Alternative Medicine Emerges in the Nation's Capital. *Advances: The Journal of Mind-Body Health* 10: 68–74.

Moyers, B. 1993. *Healing and the Mind.* New York: Doubleday.

Murphy, K. 1996. Organic Food Makers Reap Green Yields of Revenue. *New York Times* 26 October: 21, 23.

Murray, M., and Pizzorno, J. 1989. *Textbook of Natural Medicine.* Seattle, WA: John Bastyr College Publications.

Muscat, M. 1995. Message Therapy to be Licensed in Tennessee. *Alternative Therapies* 1(5): 23.

Naparstek, B. 1994. *Staying Well with Guided Imagery.* New York: Time Warner Books.

National Health Federation. n.d. Membership brochure.

National Health Federation. 1995. *Health Freedom News.*

Nebelkopf, E. 1995. Psychedelic and Shamanistic Influences in the Human Services in the U.S. *Yearbook of Cross-Cultural Medicine and Psychotherapy* 6:163–181.

New Age Journal. 1995–1996. Holistic Health Directory and Resource Guide.

New York Times. 1996. Oxford Health Plans to Cover Alternative Care. 9 October: A11.

NIH Technology Assessment Panel. 1996. Integration of Behavioral and Relaxation Approaches into the Treatment of Chronic Pain and Insomnia. *Journal of the American Medical Association* 276: 313–318.

Noonan, P. 1995. Feel Better Than You Ever Thought Possible . . . With Ayurveda. *For Women First* 4 September: 10–17.

Numbers, R. 1976. *Prophetess of Health: A Study of Ellen G. White*. New York: Harper and Row.

Oboler, S. K., and F. M. Laforce. 1989. The Periodic Physical Examination in Asymptomatic Adults. *Annals of Internal Medicine* 110: 214–226.

O'Connor, B. B. 1995. *Healing Traditions: Alternative Medicine and the Health Professions*. Philadelphia: University of Pennsylvania Press.

Office of Alternative Medicine. 1992. Workshop on Alternative Medicine. *Alternative Medicine: Expanding Medical Horizons—A Report to the National Institutes of Health in Alternative Medical Systems and Practices in the United States*. Washington, DC: U.S. Government Printing Office.

Office of Alternative Medicine. 1994. FDA to Review Status of Acupuncture Needles. *Complementary and Alternative Medicine at the NIH* 1(4): 1.

Office of Alternative Medicine. 1995. New Director Outlines Office Mission and Accomplishments. *Complementary and Alternative Medicine at the NIH* 2(5/6): 1, 4–5.

Office of Alternative Medicine. 1997. In the News. *Complementary and Alternative Medicine at the NIH* 4(4).

Office of Alternative Medicine. 1998. List of currently funded centers available at URL *http: //altmed.od.nih.gov/oam/resources/present/oam-core/* (visited 3/20/98).

Office of Technology Assessment, U.S. Congress. 1978. *Assessing the Safety and Efficacy of Medical Technologies*. Washington, DC: U.S. Congress, OTA-H-75.

Oldham, J. 1995. A Profitable Age. *Los Angeles Times* 4 July: D1.

Olmos, D. R. 1997. HMO to Offer Acupuncture; It May Be First in State to Do So. *Los Angeles Times* 23 April: D1.

Omega Institute for Holistic Studies. 1997. *Program Guide*. Rhinebeck, NY.

Ornish, D. 1990. *Dr. Dean Ornish's Program for Reversing Heart Disease*. New York: Random House.

Ornish, D. 1995. Healing the Heart, Reversing the Disease. *Alternative Therapies* 1(5): 84–92.

Oxman, T., D. Freeman, and E. Manheimer. 1995. Lack of Social Participation or Religious Strength and Comfort as Risk Factors for Death After Cardiac Surgery in the Elderly. *Psychosomatic Medicine* 57: 5–15.

Pachter, L. 1994. Culture and Clinical Care. *Journal of the American Medical Association* 271: 690–694.

Palmer, B. J. 1917. *The Science of Chiropractic* (3rd ed.). Davenport, IA: Palmer School of Chiropractic.

Palmer, D. D. 1992. *The Chiropractor's Adjuster.* Davenport, IA: Palmer College Press.

Park, R. L., and U. Goodenough. 1996. Buying Snake Oil with Tax Dollars. *New York Times* 3 January: A11.

Payer, L. 1988. *Medicine and Culture: Varieties of Treatment in the United States, England and France.* New York: Henry Holt and Company.

Pear, R. 1998. Spending on Health Grew Slowly in 1996. *New York Times* 13 January: A9.

Pelletier, K. 1979. *Holistic Medicine: From Stress to Optimum Health.* New York: Delacorte Press.

Pew Research Center for the People and the Press. 1996. *The Diminishing Divide: American Churches, American Politics.* URL *http://www.people-press.org/* (visited 8/16/97).

Pinkerton, J. P. 1996. Be Careful of Criticizing Spirituality. *New York Times* 28 June: B9.

Poloma, M. M. 1991. A Comparison of Christian Science and Mainline Christian Healing Ideologies and Practices. *Review of Religious* 32: 337–350.

Porter, J. E. 1995. OAM Funding: A Shared Responsibility. *Alternative Therapies* 1(3): 80.

Price, L. 1984. Art, Science, Faith and Medicine: The Implications of the Placebo Effect. *Sociology of Health and Illness* 6: 61–73.

Professional Association of Traditional Healers (PATH). 1996. Press release. Denver, CO. 14 October.

Quackwatch. 1998. Be Wary of "Alternative" Health Methods. Homepage. URL *http://www.quackwatch.com* (visited 3/19/98).

Rasanen, J., et al. 1996. Religious Affiliation and All Course Mortality: A Perspective Population Study in Middle-Aged Men in Eastern Finland. *International Journal of Epidemiology* 25: 1244–1249.

RB Distribution. 1996. Natural Sex. Flyer. Santa Monica, CA.

Rees, B. L. 1993. An Exploratory Study of the Effectiveness of a Relaxation With Guided Imagery Protocol. *Journal of Holistic Nursing* 11: 271–276.

Reilly, D., et al. 1994. Is Evidence for Homeopathy Reproducible? *Lancet* 334: 1601–1606.

Relman, A. 1981. Informing the Public—With Facts and Folktales. *New England Journal of Medicine* 304: 108–109.

Remen, R. N. 1992. Your Emotions and Your Health. *Unity* 172: 48–54.

Research Center for Alternative Medicine. 1997. Homepage. URL *http://www.ream.cadvision.com* (visited 8/16/97).

Reuters. 1997a. Friends and Faith Improve Cancer Odds. URL *http://www.yahoo.com/headlines/970312/health/stories* (visited 3/12/97).

Reuters. 1997b. Attitude to Exercise Affects Health. *http://www.yahoo.com/headlines/971030/health/stories* (visited 10/30/97).

Ring, K. 1980. *Life at Death: A Scientific Investigation of the Near-Death Experience.* New York: Coward, McCann and Geoghegan.

Roan, S. 1996. Rethinking Approaches to Pain Relief. *Los Angeles Times* 1 October: E1.

Robbins, T., and D. Anthony. 1979. Sociology of Contemporary Religious Movements. *Annual Review of Sociology* 5: 79–89.

Rodale Press. 1996. Press Kit for *Prevention* Magazine. Emmaus, PA.

Rolf, I. F. 1977. *The Integration of Human Structures.* Santa Monica, CA: Dennis Landman.

Rosa, L., E. Rosa, L. Sarner, and S. Barrett. 1998. A Closer Look at Therapeutic Touch. *Journal of the American Medical Association* 279: 1005–1010.

Rosenthal, E. 1991. Hands-On Back Therapy Is Winning Respectability. *New York Times* 3 July: A1, B6.

Rossman, M. 1989. *Healing Yourself: A Step by Step Program for Better Health Through Imagery.* New York: Pocket Books.

Roter, D., et al. 1997. Communication Patterns of Primary Care Physicians. *Journal of the American Medical Association* 277: 350–356.

R Pure Aloe International. n.d. A to Z: Why Aloe Vera? Pamphlet. Northglenn, CO.

Sale, D. M. 1995. *Overview of Legislative Developments Concerning Alternative Health Care in the United States.* A Research Project of the Fetzer Institute.

Salmon, J. W., and Berliner, H. S. 1980. Health Policy Implications of the Holistic Health Movement. *Journal of Health Politics, Policy and Law* 5: 535–553.

Samuels, M., and H. Bennet. 1973. *The Well-Body Book.* New York: Random House.

Sapolsky, R. M. 1990. Stress in the Wild. *Scientific American* 262: 116–123.

Schnall, P. L., et al. 1990. The Relationship Between "Job Strain," Workplace Diastolic Blood Pressure, and Left Ventricular Mass Index: Results of a Case Control Study. *Journal of the American Medical Association* 263: 1929–1935.

Schneider, E. L., and J. M. Guralnik. 1990. The Aging of America: Impact on Health Care Costs. *Journal of the American Medical Association* 263: 2335–2340.

Schwartz, H. 1986. *Never Satisfied: A Cultural History of Diets, Fantasies, and Fat.* New York: The Free Press.

Seligman, J., and G. Cowley. 1995. Sex, Lies and Garlic. *Newsweek* 6 November: 65–68.

Selye, H. 1956. *The Stress of Life.* New York: McGraw Hill.

Shapiro, D. H., and R. N. Walsh. 1984. *Meditation: Classical and Contemporary Perspectives.* New York: Aldine.

Shapiro, D. H., et al. 1997. Reduction in Drug Requirements for Hypertension by Means of Cognitive-Behavioral Intervention. *American Journal of Hypertension* 10: 9–17.

Sharma, H. M., B. D. Triguna, and D. Chopra. 1991. Maharishi Ayur-Veda: Modern Insights into Ancient Medicine. *Journal of the American Medical Association* 265: 2633–2637.

Sharma, U. 1992. *Complementary Medicine Today: Practitioners and Patients.* London and New York: Tavistock/Routledge.

Shealy, C. N., and C. Myss. 1993. *The Creation of Health.* Walpole, NH: Stillpoint Publications.

Shekelle, P. G. 1994. Spine Update—Spinal Manipulation. *Spine* 1980: 858–861.

Simonton, O. C., S. Matthews-Simonton, and J. L. Creighton. 1978. *Getting Well Again.* New York: Bantam Books.

Skolnick, A. A. 1991. Maharishi's Ayur-Veda: Guru's Marketing Scheme Promises the World Eternal "Perfect Health." *Journal of the American Medical Association* 266: 1741–1750.

Smith, M. E. G. 1992. The Burzynski Controversy in the United States and Canada: A Comparative Case Study in the Sociology of Alternative Medicine. *Canadian Journal of Sociology* 17: 133–159.

Sobel, D. S. 1995. Rethinking Medicine: Improving Health Outcomes with Cost-Effective Psychosocial Interventions. *Psychosomatic Medicine* 57: 234–244.

Spencer, J., and W. Jonas. 1997. And Now, Alternative Medicine. *Archives of Family Medicine* 6: 155–156.

Starr, P. 1982. *The Social Transformation of American Medicine.* New York: Basic Books.

Stawbridge, W., et al. 1997. Frequent Attendance of Religious Services and Mortality Over 28 Years. *American Journal of Public Health* 87: 957–961.

Stevenson, C. 1995. Non-pharmacological Aspects of Acute Pain Management. *Complementary Therapies in Nurse Midwifery* 1: 77–84.

Struna, N. 1981. Sport and Colonial Education: A Cultural Perspective. *Research Quarterly for Exercise and Sport* 52: 117–135.

Szasz, T. 1975. *Ceremonial Chemistry.* Garden City, NY: Doubleday Anchor.

Thomson, B. 1996. The Medical Revolution. *Natural Health* March/April: 98–103.

Tierra, L. 1992. *The Herbs of Life: Health and Healing Using Western and Chinese Techniques.* Freedom, CA: The Crossing Press.

Todd, A. D. 1994. *Double Vision: An East-West Collaboration for Coping with Cancer.* Hanover, NH: Wesleyan University Press/University Press of New England.

Tovey, P. 1997. Contingent Legitimacy: U.K. Alternative Practitioners and Intersectoral Acceptance. *Social Science and Medicine* 45: 1129–1133.

Trachtman, P. 1994. NIH Looks at the Implausible and the Inexplicable. *Smithsonian* September: 110–124.

Turner, B. 1982. The Government of the Body: Medical Regimens and the Rationalization of Diet. *British Journal of Sociology* 33: 254–269.

Turner, R. 1992. Ideology and Utopia After Socialism. Pp. 79–100 in *New Social Movements: From Ideology to Identity.* Edited by E. Laraña, H. Johnston, and J. Gusfield. Philadelphia: Temple University Press.

Turner, S. 1995. Taking Health to Heart. *Hospitals and Health Networks* 69: 79–80.

Ullman, D. 1986. *Strategies for Making Alternative Health Part of the Progressive's Health Care Agenda.* Berkeley, CA: Homeopathic Educational Services.

Ullman, D. 1991. *Discovering Homeopathy: Your Introduction to The Science and Art of Homeopathic Medicine.* Berkeley, CA: North Atlantic Books.

U.S. Bureau of the Census. *Statistical Abstract of the United States: 1996* (116th ed.). Washington, D.C.

Vanderpool, H. 1984. The Holistic Hodgepodge: A Critical Analysis. *Journal of Family Practice* 19: 773–781.

van Gelder, L. 1996. Thomas S. Kuhn: Scholar Who Altered the Paradigm of Scientific Change Dies at 73. *New York Times* 19 February: B9.

Villaire, M. 1995. OAM Report. *Alternative Therapies* 1(1): 10–11.

Vishnudevananda, S. 1980. *The Complete Illustrated Book of Yoga.* New York: Harmony Books.

Walker, M. 1990. *The Chelation Way.* Garden City Park, NY: Avery Publishing Group, Inc.

Walker, M. 1995. *Jumping for Health.* Garden City Park, NY: Avery Publishing Group, Inc.

Wallis, C. 1991. The New Age of Alternative Medicine. *Time Magazine* 4 November: 68–76.

Wallis, C. 1996. Faith and Healing. *Time Magazine* 24 June: 58–64.

Walters, R. 1993. *Options: The Alternative Cancer Therapy Book*. Garden City Park, NY: Avery Publishing Group, Inc.

Watson, J. 1995. Nursing's Caring—Healing Paradigm: An Exemplar for Alternative Medicine? *Alternative Therapies* 1(3): 64.

Weeks, N. 1973. *The Medical Discoveries of Edward Bach, Physician*. London: C. W. Daniel Co.

Weil, A. 1988. *Health and Healing*. Boston: Houghton Mifflin.

Weil, A. 1997a. *Eight Weeks to Optimum Health: A Proven Program for Taking Full Advantage of Your Body's Natural Healing Power*. New York: Knopf.

Weil, A. 1997b. Ask Dr. Weil. Homepage of Andrew Weil. URL *http: //cgi. pathfinder.com/drweil/home* (visited 3/7/97, 9/19/97).

Weil, A., and W. Rosen 1993. *Chocolate to Morphine: Understanding Drugs*. Boston: Houghton Mifflin.

Wennberg, J. E. 1984. Dealing With Medical Practice Variations: A Proposal for Action. *Health Affairs* 3: 3–62.

Werbach, M. R. 1986. *Third Line Medicine*. New York: Arkana.

Wetzel, M. S., Eisenberg, D. M., and T. J. Kaptchuk. 1998. Courses Involving Complementary and Alternative Medicine at U.S. Medical Schools. *Journal of the American Medical Association* 280: 784–787.

Whole Life Expo 1996. Program guide. Pasadena, CA. 15 March.

Whorton, J. 1982. *Crusaders for Fitness: The History of American Health Reformers*. Princeton, NJ: Princeton University Press.

Williams S. 1997. Modern Medicine and the Uncertain Body: From Corporeality to Hyperreality. *Social Science and Medicine* 45: 1041–1049.

Williams S. J., and M. Calnan. 1996. The "Limits" of Medicalization?: Modern Medicine and the Lay Populace in "Late" Modernity. *Social Science and Medicine* 42(12): 1609–1620.

Wolfe, B. L. 1986. Health Status and Medical Expenditures: Is There a Link? *Social Science and Medicine* 22: 993–999.

Wolpe, P. R. 1990. The Holistic Heresy: Strategies of Ideological Challenge. *Social Science and Medicine* 31: 913–923.

Woolhandler, S., and D. U. Himmelstein. 1997. Costs of Care and Administration at For-Profit and Other Hospitals in the U. S. *New England Journal of Medicine* 336: 769–774.

Wuthnow, R. 1997. *The Crisis in Churches: Spiritual Malaise, Fiscal Woe*. New York: Oxford University Press.

Yates, P. M., et al. 1993. Patients With Terminal Cancer Who Use Alternative Therapies: Their Beliefs and Practices. *Sociology of Health and Illness* 15: 199–216.

Yoga Journal. 1997. Webwatch. January/February.

Young, H. 1961. *The Toadstool Millionaires: A Social History of Patent Medicine in America Before Regulation*. Princeton, NJ: Princeton University Press.

Zachariae, R., et al. 1994. Changes in Cellular Immune Function After Immune Specific Guided Imagery and Relaxation in High and Low Hypnotizable Healthy Subjects. *Psychotherapy and Psychosomatics* 61: 74–95.

Zola, I. 1978. Medicine as an Institution of Social Control. Pp. 80–101 in *The Cultural Crisis of Modern Medicine*. Edited by J. Ehrenreich. New York: Monthly Review Press.

Zwicky J. F., et al. 1993. *Reader's Guide to Alternative Methods: An Analysis of More than 1,000 Reports on Unproven, Disproven, Controversial, Fraudulent, Quack, and/or Otherwise Questionable Approaches to Solving Health Problems*. Chicago, IL: American Medical Association.

Index

essential careers™

A CAREER AS AN
AUTO
MECHANIC

TAMRA B. ORR

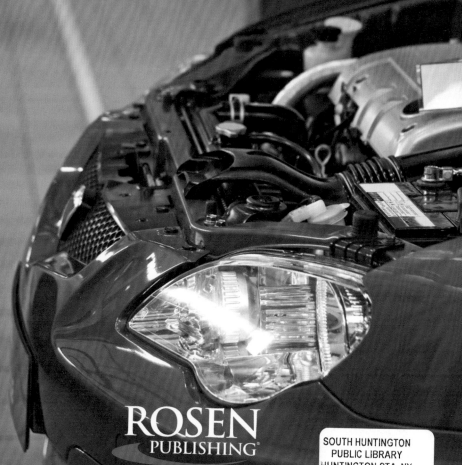

ROSEN
PUBLISHING®

NEW YORK

Published in 2011 by The Rosen Publishing Group, Inc.
29 East 21st Street, New York, NY 10010

Copyright © 2011 by The Rosen Publishing Group, Inc.

First Edition

Library of Congress Cataloging-in-Publication Data

Orr, Tamra B.
A career as an auto mechanic / Tamra B. Orr.—1st ed.
    p. cm.—(Essential careers)
Includes bibliographical references and index.
ISBN 978-1-4358-9471-6 (library binding)
1. Automobiles—Maintenance and repair—Juvenile literature. 2. Automobile mechanics—Vocational guidance—Juvenile literature. I. Title.
TL152.O77 2011
629.28'72023—dc22

                                                                2009046608

Manufactured in the United States of America

CPSIA Compliance Information: Batch #S10YA: For further information, contact Rosen Publishing, New York, New York, at 1-800-237-9932.

contents

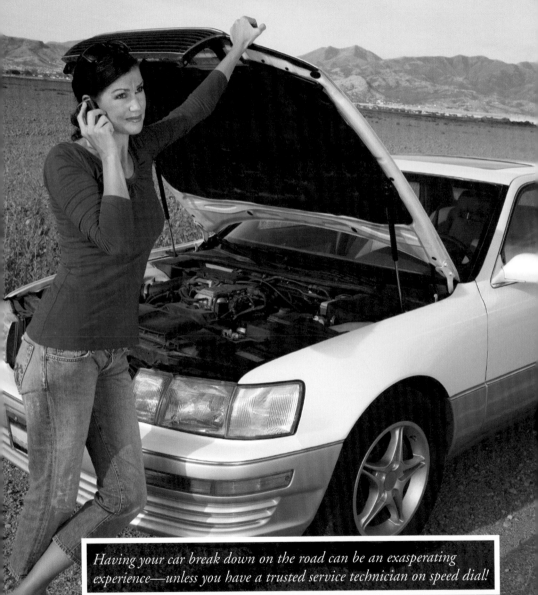

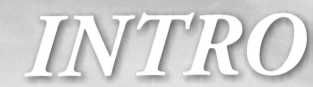
INTRO

Having your car break down on the road can be an exasperating experience—unless you have a trusted service technician on speed dial!

DUCTION

There is an old saying that goes, "You don't know what you've got till it's gone." Similarly, it might be said that, "You don't know what you've got till it doesn't work." This is certainly true when it comes to any kind of vehicle—from cars to trucks, motorcycles to airplanes, buses to boats, semitrailers to trains. North Americans are extremely dependent on their nations' transportation systems and the machines and vehicles used to get from one place to another.

Every day, people depend on vehicles of various kinds to get to work, school, friends' houses, the store, and then back home again. Most people take it for granted that when they turn the key or take a seat, the vehicle they are in will start—and go! Sometimes, however, it doesn't. A crucial part fails, falls apart, or wears out. Suddenly a routine trip becomes a voyage to nowhere. The first reaction is often to run, not walk, to the nearest mechanic who can figure out the problem and fix it.

The first car was invented in 1886. The first paved road was constructed in 1903. And ever since these key dates, a mechanic who could figure out which part of a vehicle was not working and then fix it properly was in high demand.

Although cars and every other type of motorized vehicle have changed dramatically over the last century, the demand for qualified and skilled mechanics—better known today as service technicians—has only grown. The job has gotten more difficult over the years as cars and trucks have become far more technologically complex. Engines and "onboard" systems now include computer chips and electronic gadgetry never dreamed of when

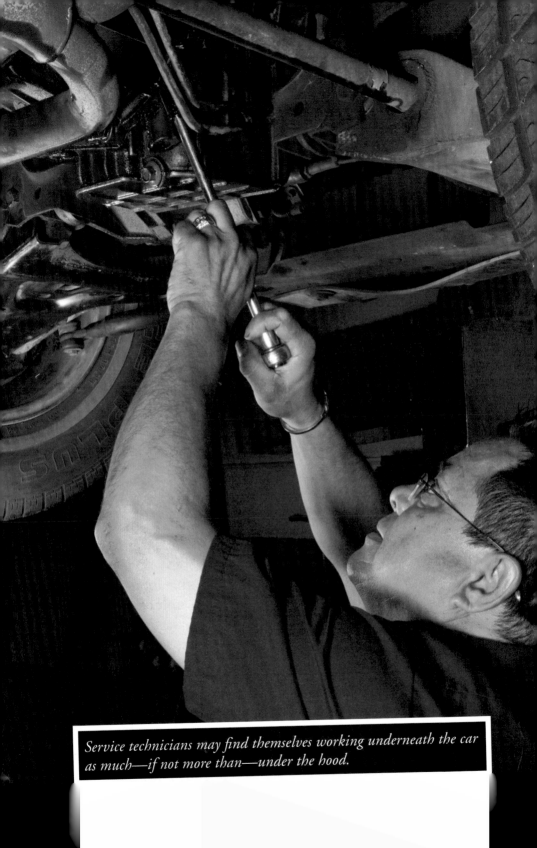

Service technicians may find themselves working underneath the car as much—if not more than—under the hood.

Henry Ford was designing the technological marvels of his age—the Model T car and the assembly lines that would rapidly produce it in great numbers. As consumers and manufacturers become more "green" and vehicles shift to engines powered by alternative fuels, the knowledge, practical skill, and experience a technician will need to possess will only increase.

Most professions are negatively affected when the economy undergoes a crisis like a severe recession. Yet the maintenance and repair of engines and other equipment is work that remains in demand, even when consumer interest in other goods and services slackens and money is tight. During good economic times, consumers buy new equipment that requires regular maintenance and occasional repair. During the lean economic times, they want to keep what they have in the best possible working condition so that they won't have to replace it. This, too, requires regular maintenance and repair.

A knowledgeable and trustworthy service technician is valued and needed in today's transportation-centered world. A person may choose to focus on working with personal vehicles like cars, motorcycles, or boats, or with larger passenger vehicles like airplanes or trains, or even with small engines like lawn mowers or chainsaws. Regardless of the specialty, there will almost certainly be work for mechanics wherever they go and whatever their area of expertise.

The field of mechanics is vast, as are the job opportunities, career paths, and areas of specialization. It's an exciting field that is just right for people who like to get their hands dirty—literally. It's a profession for those who believe in old-fashioned hand tools coupled with tomorrow's most sophisticated computer and electronic systems. Most importantly, it's the ideal field for those who love to take things apart, figure out how something should work and why it doesn't, identify and fix the problem, and put the machine back together again, now running better than ever.

chapter 1

BREAKDOWN!

Every driver has been through it at least once: the engine that just will not start or cranks but won't turn over. There is the "check engine" light that keeps flashing red every time you turn on the ignition. Then there is the dead battery, the brakes that squeal, or the high-pitched whine of a loose fan belt. The clutch slips, or the idle is too fast or slow. These are inevitable moments for anyone who owns any kind of machine that houses an engine.

Many people, unfortunately, have also found themselves in a fender bender or other vehicular accident that means something—or possibly everything—on a car or truck has to be fixed. With an average of six million auto accidents each year in the United States, it seems almost inevitable that everyone will have a crunch or crash at some point and their car will have to go into the shop.

AUTO TECHNICIAN TO THE RESCUE

Every day, the United States' 4 million miles (6,437,376 kilometers) of roads, streets, and highways are filled with 136 million passenger cars, 7 million motorcycles, and more than 2 million trucks. Every kind of vehicle—from the passenger car

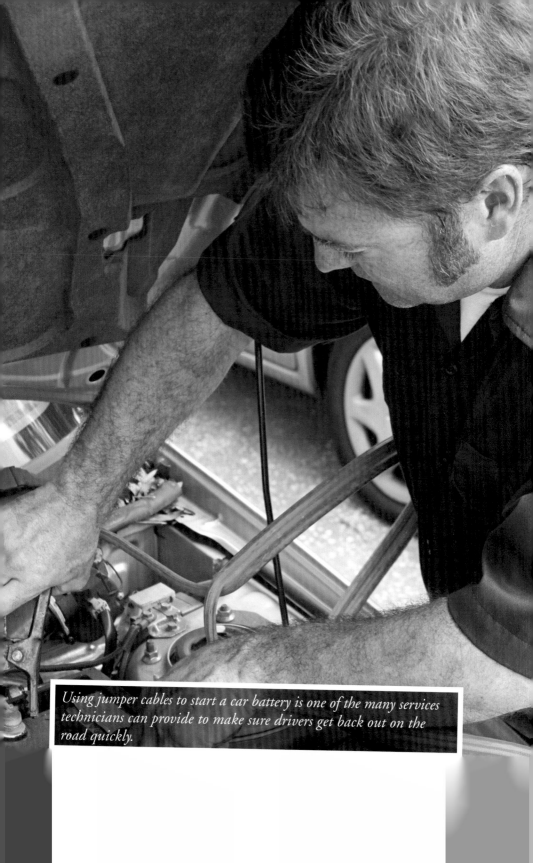

Using jumper cables to start a car battery is one of the many services technicians can provide to make sure drivers get back out on the road quickly.

and the jet plane to the motor scooter and the cabin cruiser—is full of hundreds of moving parts. These will need to be maintained, repaired, and replaced on a regular basis.

That is where the mechanic, or service technician, enters the picture. This is the person who can do with vehicles what a good physician can do with bodies. He or she tests to make sure all of the parts are running the way they are designed to. The service technician diagnoses any problems. Broken or malfunctioning parts are either repaired or replaced. Today's technician can be found working in small garages and shops, service stations, large car dealerships, or even the military. Some also work in auto parts stores, tire stores, vehicle leasing companies, or equipment rental businesses, or with organizations like the American Automobile Association (AAA). Technicians are typically responsible for inspecting, maintaining, and repairing a variety of vehicles. These vehicles have engines or motors that run on gasoline, electricity, a combination of both, or alternative fuels.

A DAY ON THE JOB

There is really no such thing as a typical day for an auto mechanic, and this is one of the great joys of the job. Depending on where the technician works, he or she may be rebuilding an engine one moment and changing spark plugs the next. The mechanic may go from repairing a front axle to replacing an air filter. He or she may work on foreign models or domestic—or both. He or she may be diagnosing the problem on an air-cooled 1977 Volkswagen bus one day and repairing the self-parking mechanism on a Lexus LS 460 the next. Everything depends on what kind of mechanic the person is, what model cars his or her shop or dealership specializes in, and what the area of expertise is.

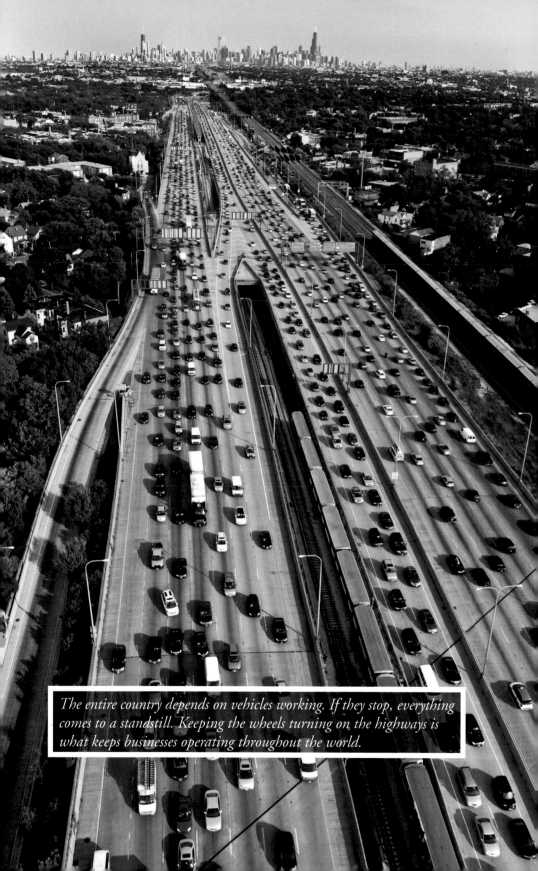

The entire country depends on vehicles working. If they stop, everything comes to a standstill. Keeping the wheels turning on the highways is what keeps businesses operating throughout the world.

The tools used on the job will vary greatly, from old-fashioned hand tools and grease and oil, to power tools and diagnostic computers. In a large dealership garage or chain service center, such as Goodwrench, Midas, or Jiffy Lube, the mechanic may start his or her day by reporting to a service manager. He or she will decide which of the many vehicles to begin working on. Or in a smaller shop, the mechanic may chat with the customer to find out what seems to be wrong with the car and then go for a test drive to further diagnose the problem. Then the mechanic would begin working on the car and fixing what was wrong. The unpredictability of the job, of course, is one of its advantages. It keeps the work interesting and makes every day different from the one before it. It also ensures that the mechanic keeps up to date on the latest models, the newest techniques, and the most reliable repairs.

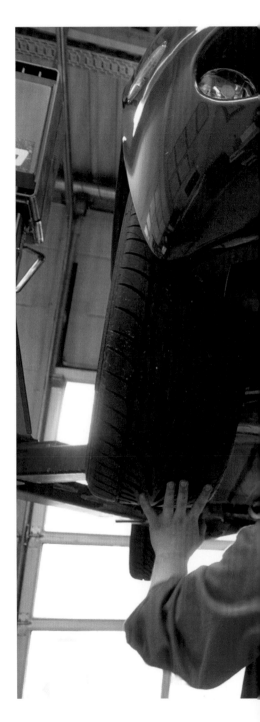

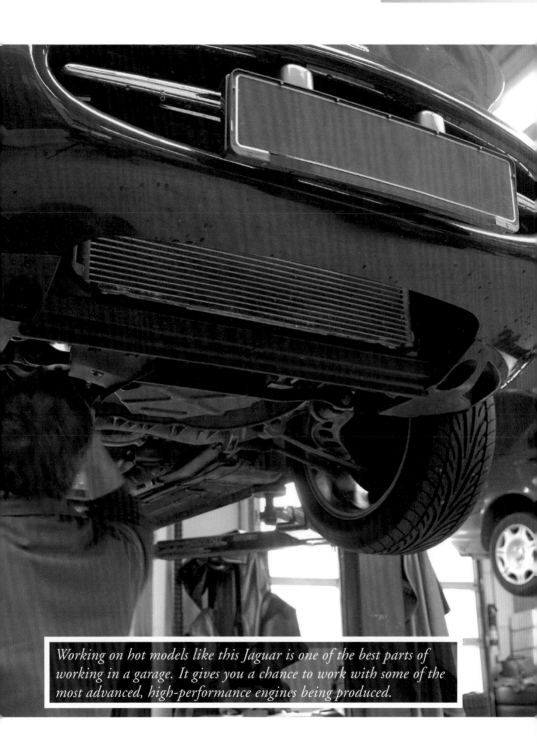

Working on hot models like this Jaguar is one of the best parts of working in a garage. It gives you a chance to work with some of the most advanced, high-performance engines being produced.

DIAGNOSING AND FIXING THE PROBLEM

Diagnosing what is wrong with a vehicle is often tricky, just like determining what is wrong when a person is ill. There are so

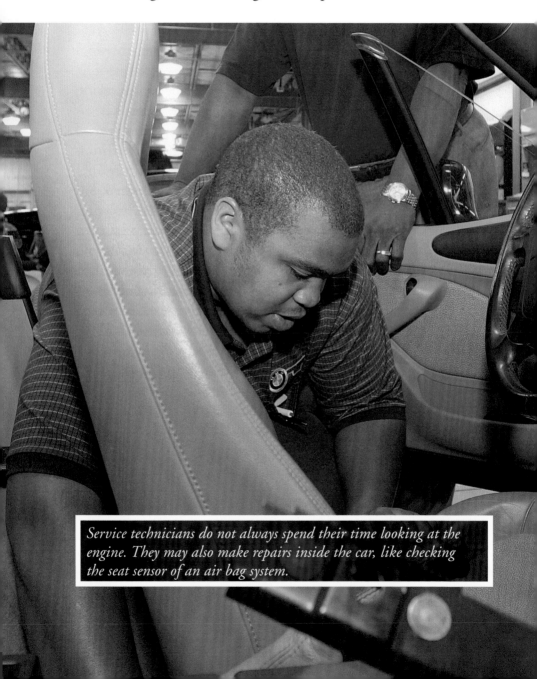

Service technicians do not always spend their time looking at the engine. They may also make repairs inside the car, like checking the seat sensor of an air bag system.

many auto parts that can malfunction that it can be challenging to figure out which one is performing badly and why. It frequently takes a combination of years of practical experience, old-fashioned "elbow grease" working with hand tools, computerized diagnostics, and a sharp set of eyes and ears to figure it all out.

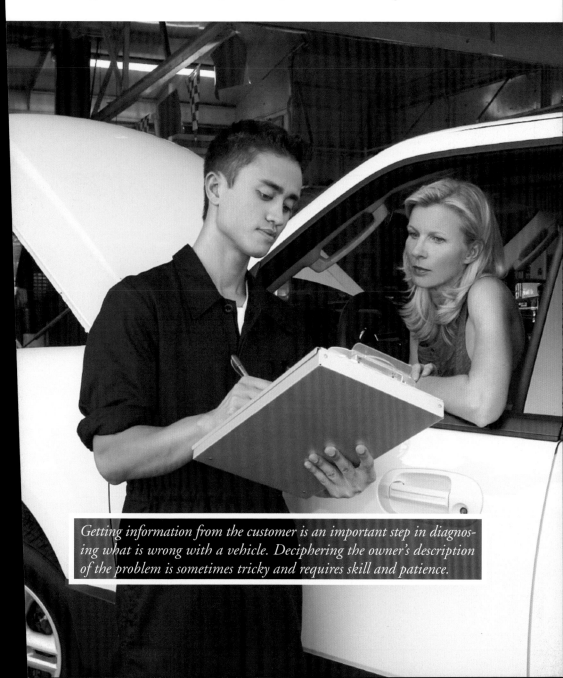

Getting information from the customer is an important step in diagnosing what is wrong with a vehicle. Deciphering the owner's description of the problem is sometimes tricky and requires skill and patience.

Although the mechanic may get some valuable information from customers, more often than not they tend to describe problems in vague terms, like "sputter," "ping," or "buzz." These kinds of descriptions rarely pinpoint a problem, but they may still provide a few clues. So it's important to listen to customers, even if their mechanical knowledge is lacking.

Once the diagnosis has been made on a car, it's time to decide what to do about it. Again, effective auto repair requires years of practical experience and mechanical knowledge to determine not only what to fix or replace, but also how to go about doing it properly. If new parts are needed,

THE *CAR TALK* GUYS

There are few people who have made auto mechanics as fun—and funny—as the siblings Tom and Ray Magliozzi, better known as Click and Clack, the Tappet Brothers. They are the hosts of the show *Car Talk* on National Public Radio. Since 1987, they have been entertaining listeners by taking phone-in questions about car problems and seeing if they can find possible solutions on the air. The brothers typically attract more than four million listeners on six hundred radio stations nationwide. In addition to their show, the duo have authored books, created an award-winning Web site, and written a column published in more than three hundred newspapers.

Together, Click and Clack have a great deal of experience with cars, having run their own car repair service for years. Coupled with their thick Boston accents, degrees from the Massachusetts Institute of Technology (MIT), and wisecracking banter, they keep people entertained and educated about car care.

the technician will often have to contact a variety of parts suppliers to find the right part for the right price. The cost of parts is added to the expected cost of the labor (usually a per-hour charge), and that price is given to the customer for approval. This price is known as an estimate. If the customer agrees to the proposed price of the repair, work can begin.

Of course, not all the work that mechanics do is repairs. Many technicians spend their days performing routine maintenance and inspections. They typically follow a checklist of what to examine, such as belts, hoses, plugs, brakes, the fuel

THE MOST COMMON CAR TROUBLES

There are countless things that can go wrong with an automobile, but some are far more common than others. Some car parts wear out faster because they get more use. Here are the ten areas that car service technicians must repair the most often:

1. Brake system
2. Engine lubrication (oil changes) and air filters
3. Radiator
4. Ignition or electronic control
5. Steering/suspension
6. Carburetor/fuel system
7. Electrical system
8. Transmission/clutch/rear axle
9. Climate control (air-conditioning, heating, and defrosting)
10. Exhaust system

and exhaust systems, and tires. This helps prevent major break-downs and repairs "down the road."

Once the work on a car is finished, technicians may take the vehicle for a test drive and then let the customer know the job is done. The work usually does not stop there, however. Now it's time for cleaning the bay and tools and getting ready for the next car in line outside the garage.

Being a service technician can be a fascinating job. It constantly changes with the times and with each technological advance. New skills must always be acquired and new mechanical challenges met with each new model of car that rolls off the assembly line. Auto repair and maintenance is work that people will always need, no matter the direction technology may take.

chapter 2

GETTING A HEAD START

E ven though you may still be a student in high school, you do not have to wait to get started in the field of automotive service. There are a number of steps you can take right now that will give you a head start later on when you either pursue further education or begin looking for a job.

ASK YOURSELF THIS

First of all, do an inventory of the skills and interests you already have. Ask yourself a few questions, such as:

1. Do I like to work with my hands?
2. What power/machine/hand tools do I already know how to use?
3. Do I enjoy taking things apart and putting them back together again?
4. Do I get a sense of satisfaction from taking something that isn't working, locating the problem, and repairing it?
5. What do I already know about engines and how they work?
6. What experience have I had so far working with different types of vehicles?
7. Do I prefer working alone or with others?

8. Is there anyone I know who works as a mechanic whom I could interview, shadow, or ask to be my mentor?
9. Do I have a favorite make, model, style, or type of vehicle that I would like to work with more than others?

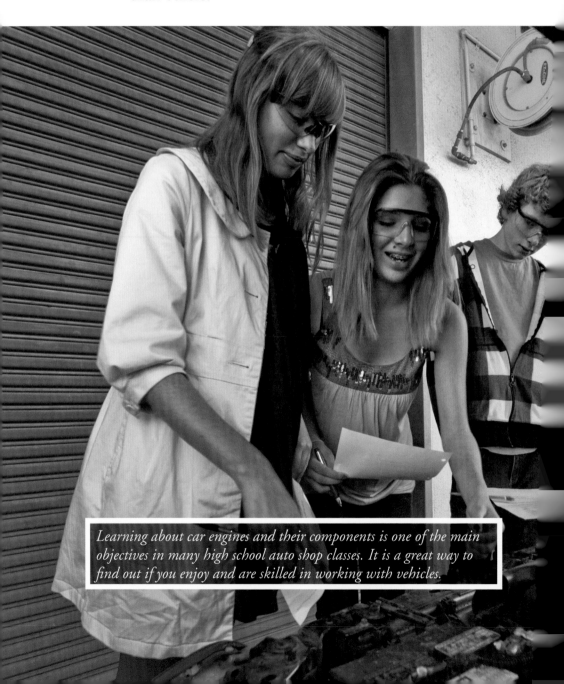

Learning about car engines and their components is one of the main objectives in many high school auto shop classes. It is a great way to find out if you enjoy and are skilled in working with vehicles.

10. Do I prefer working with vintage cars, high-performance sports cars, or the latest models? Do I prefer working on foreign models or American cars?
11. What vocational and community colleges are in my area that might be able to offer further information?

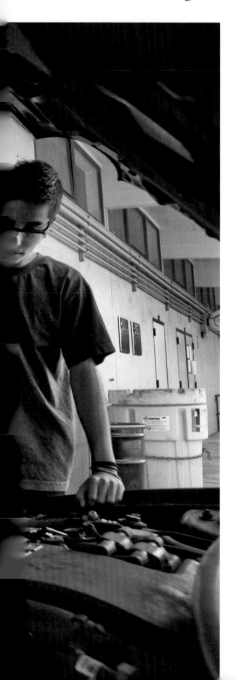

12. How strong is my background in math, physics, electronics, mechanical engineering, and computers?

Once you have answered these questions, you will have a clearer vision of where you are starting from, where you want to go, and how to get there.

RESEARCHING THE FIELD

The next step is to do your homework. Act as if your interest in automotive care is a homework assignment or research paper and start studying the field. There are several things you can do to begin familiarizing yourself with the auto care industry and the necessary educational preparation.

Search the Internet to see what you can find out about educational programs, standard certification tests, and potential internships. There are hundreds of sites to

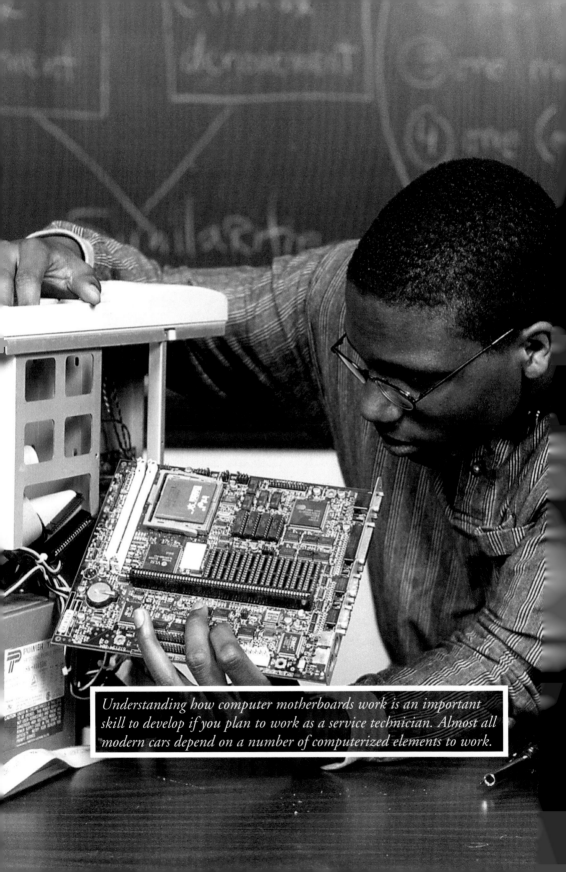

Understanding how computer motherboards work is an important skill to develop if you plan to work as a service technician. Almost all modern cars depend on a number of computerized elements to work.

explore on the topic. Stop by both school and public libraries to see what books and other resource materials they have to offer. They frequently have automotive how-to books and videos available to loan.

WELL-ROUNDED SKILLS AND KNOWLEDGE

"Having the skills and ability to utilize today's technology in automotive repair is crucial for anyone entering into this field. Vehicles are highly computerized, and being comfortable working with computers and scanning tools is a must for anyone entering this field. Service information, for the most part, is now all computerized. This is not a 'learn this instead of that' kind of proposal. This is now the minimum you need to enter this industry. These skills must be strong and combined with automotive-specific knowledge. The two areas need to work together to determine the root cause of what is wrong with a vehicle.

"Students should try to keep their background as well-rounded as they can. Automotive technicians need to obviously have automotive and computer skills, but also be able to use logic, computer programming, and systematic approaches to problem solving. Being well-read and understanding new technologies and how they are applied and developed for today's vehicles are essential. Anybody going into automotive repair should be familiar with the government regulations.

"Also technicians must be high-tech adapters. The technology is changing daily. Gone are the days of the grease monkey and a service manual. Today's techs use social networking sites to share experiences and solve problems with fellow mechanics."—*Art Jacobsen, director of business development for CarMD*

If there is a local car garage that has caught your eye, go in and see if you can chat with the owner for a few minutes about his or her business. Stop by a dealership that sells your favorite brand of car and ask if you can interview a couple of the mechanics. Be prepared for them to say yes and have your questions written out and ready to go, just in case. These are busy workers, and you don't want to take up too much of their time.

Ask your guidance counselor about any internships or apprenticeships that he or she is aware of in the area. Explore the vocational schools and community colleges in your region. What courses, certification, and degree programs do they offer? What are the academic requirements, course times, and cost?

Read the local ads in the newspaper and see if any garages or instructors are offering noncredit, community courses in mechanics. Can you take some of these classes now while you are still in high school? Keep an eye out for ads and opportunities that are not necessarily focused exclusively on cars but on small engines, too, such as a class in repairing lawn mowers or garden tractors. Perhaps someone is offering a weekend class on fixing boat engines or motorcycle maintenance. Seize as many of these opportunities as possible. They might help you refine your interests, even as you develop solid overall mechanical skills.

Let your parents and neighbors know about your interest as well. They might know someone who can help you or at least invite you over to watch them replace a set of spark plugs or a clutch cable. Check out the bulletin boards in grocery stores, libraries, your school, city hall, and other public gathering spots. That is often where listings for small automotive and mechanics classes will be posted. If you're especially interested in a certain type of class but can't find one, why not take

THE AUTOMOTIVE MAINTENANCE MERIT BADGE

How about earning a badge from the Boy Scouts of America in automotive maintenance? It has been offered since 1992. The requirements are divided into a dozen steps. In the process of earning the badge, you will learn the function of most of the car's systems, as well as a number of skills including, but not limited to:

- Checking the levels of various fluids, such as brake fluid, engine oil, coolant, power steering fluid, windshield washer fluid, transmission fluid, and battery fluid
- Locating fuse boxes and replacing blown fuses
- Checking the tension of belts and hoses
- Locating and checking air filters
- Understanding the significance of all dashboard gauges, lights, and symbols
- Checking and inflating tires
- Understanding how different types of engines operate
- Learning how to flush and change the engine coolant
- Understanding how to change the spark plugs
- Demonstrating how to connect and use jumper cables
- Checking the condition of the brakes and making any necessary repairs
- Performing an oil change and change of oil filter
- Changing a tire with a jack
- Exploring career opportunities in the automotive industry

the time to write up what you're looking for and post it on the same bulletin boards? You might find enough like-minded people to start a class, or at least an instructor who is willing to teach you the basics.

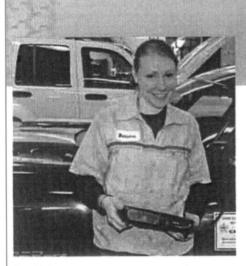

Facilities

Lab activities take place at Mercer's Auto Shop, which houses the latest tools and other equipment utilized in a typical new car dealership or auto repair shop. The Auto Shop is located at the Assunpink Campus of the Mercer County Technical Schools, across from MCCC's West Windsor Campus on Old Trenton Road.

Admission Requirements

Admission to the program requires a high school diploma or its equivalent and a strong interest in a career in automotive technology. Admission is competitive and determined based on skill levels, program-specific testing, and a personal interview with program representatives. Any required academic foundation classes should be completed before starting automotive classes.

The program may be completed in two years beginning in the fa...

required each y...

centrated two-d...

attend automoti...

Tuesdays and T...

in the afternoon...

eight-week inter...

facility.

Note: Because of the program's internship component, prospective students must be eligible to work legally in the United States to complete the degree.

Course Requirements

Curriculum

Code	Course (lecture/lab hours)	Credits
AUT 110	Introduction to Automotive Electronics (3/1)	3
AUT 111	Automotive Service Fundamentals (2/6)	5
ENG 101	English Composition I (3/0)	3
AUT 112	Automotive Fuel Systems (2/2)	3
AUT 113	Suspension, Steering and Alignment (2/4)	4
MAT 140	Applied College Algebra (4/0)[1]	4
AUT 122	Internship in Automotive Technology I	1
AUT 211	Automotive Emissions and Driveability Diagnosis (2/2)	3
AUT 212	Automotive Air Conditioning (2/2)	3
ENG 112	English Composition II with Speech (3/0)	3
AUT 115	Automotive Brake Systems (2/4)	4
AUT 114	Automotive Electricity and Electronics (2/2)	3
AUT 123	Internship in Automotive Technology II	1
HPE 110	Concepts of Health and Fitness (1/2)†	2
— —	General Education elective[2]	3
AUT 213	Engine Service (2/4)	4
AUT 221	Internship in Automotive Technology III	1
AUT 224	Manual Transmissions and Drivelines (2/3)	3
PHY 111	Physical Science Concepts (2/2)	3
AUT 222	Internship in Automotive Technology IV	1
AUT 225	Automatic Transmission Service (2/3)	3
IST 101	Computer Concepts with Applications (2/2) OR	3
IST 102	Computer Concepts with Programming (2/2)	3

General Education elective...

66

...order

NOTE...

Humanities, Historical Perspective, Diversity and Global Perspective.

†HPE 111 is an acceptable alternative.

Check out the course listings at local community colleges, like this one from Mercer County Community College in West Windsor, New Jersey. Read through the descriptions carefully to see if there are some classes you can take after school or on the weekends.

HIGH SCHOOL CLASSES

Be sure to take the appropriate classes in high school. Which ones are they? Classes in math and English are important, of course, as you will be working with both numbers and words on a daily basis. In addition, a strong background in science, including electronics, computer technology, and physics, is also helpful. Obviously, if your school offers any classes or workshops on car maintenance and repair or small engine work, take those as well. Some high schools also partner with local community colleges to create vocational technical courses. Several times a week, you may travel to the college to take a course that will earn you both high school credit and invaluable hands-on experience.

Don't sit back and wait for graduation day to begin developing your interest in automotive mechanics. Watch for opportunities all around you, and, when you spot one, grab it. These experiences will either help you decide that mechanics is not the way you want to go, or confirm that you find it fascinating, are good at it, and are eager to learn as much as you can.

:C Highlights

1ercer offers flexible scheduling for working stu-
. Many of the required academic classes can be
 in the evening or on weekends in the spring, sum-
and fall semesters.
1ercer's affordable tuition makes college possible.
 students save many thousands of dollars com-
 to costs at a four-year school. Mercer offers an
of scholarships and financial aid opportunities.
:ademic classes may be taken on either the West
or Campus or the James Kerney Campus in down-
renton. Some classes may also be taken through
s Virtual College via internet or television.
udents are Mercer's top priority. Classes are small
udents receive individual attention from a faculty
dedicated to student success. Academic advis-
reer and personal counseling, and tutoring are
le as needed.
 those who wish to pursue a career immediately
arning their associate degree, Mercer's AAS
ns are designed for direct entry into the workforce
ecific focus on job readiness.
 those interested in transferring for their bach-
egree, Mercer offers dual admissions and other
 agreements both in New Jersey and across the
. Studies show that those who transfer from a

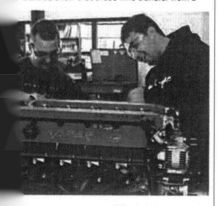

chapter 3

AFTER HIGH SCHOOL

I n the late 1960s, the automotive repair industry was under intense scrutiny. Countless complaints of fraud had been forwarded to the U.S. Congress, and the government was finally taking action. During the hearings, it was determined that the real problem was not mechanics trying to swindle customers, but mechanics who were simply not adequately trained for the job. Since there was no official way to identify and distinguish between the skilled technicians and the poorly trained ones through professional licensing or certification, customers often made the wrong choices when choosing a mechanic. Anyone with a toolbox could put out a sign saying he or she was a mechanic, but which ones could really be trusted?

Congress decided the solution was to pass a number of laws and regulations regarding the licensing of technicians. Those in the business, however, were not so sure this was the best option. Instead, the National Automobile Dealers Association and the former Motor Vehicle Manufacturers Association banded together to create the National Institute for Automotive Service Excellence (ASE).

ASE CERTIFICATION EXAMS

The purpose of the ASE was to create a set of tests that would ensure motor vehicle technicians were thoroughly

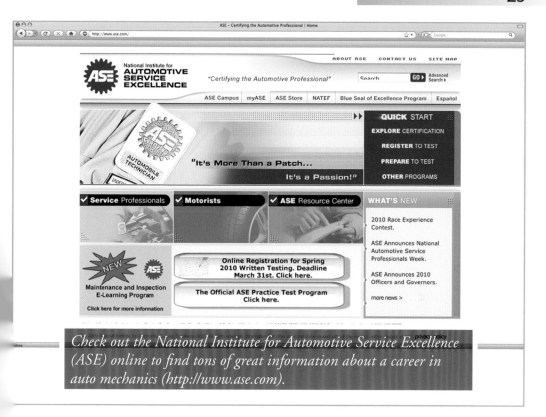

Check out the National Institute for Automotive Service Excellence (ASE) online to find tons of great information about a career in auto mechanics (http://www.ase.com).

knowledgeable in their respective fields and could earn the official certification to prove it. This could help customers distinguish the competent from the incompetent technicians by setting a basic standard. Through the ASE, dozens of tests were developed in eight primary categories of maintenance and repair:

1. Engine repair
2. Automatic transmission/transaxle
3. Manual drive train and axles
4. Suspension and steering
5. Brakes
6. Electrical/electronic systems
7. Heating and air-conditioning
8. Engine performance

Each test has between forty and eighty multiple-choice questions, many of them accompanied by detailed schematics and illustrations. When one exam is passed, the person receives a certificate and a patch denoting expertise in that skill area. If all eight tests are passed, the technician is certified as a master technician. Before each test can be taken, a technician must have worked in the field for two years, or one year plus attendance at an accredited training program. A number of preparation guides for these tests can be found in book and/or CD-ROM form, as well as on the ASE Web site.

To maintain certification, tests have to be retaken every five years. This way, the technician stays up to date on all of the changing technology that is part of the profession. These recertification tests are about half as long as the original ones. The ASE offers additional tests in the following specializations:

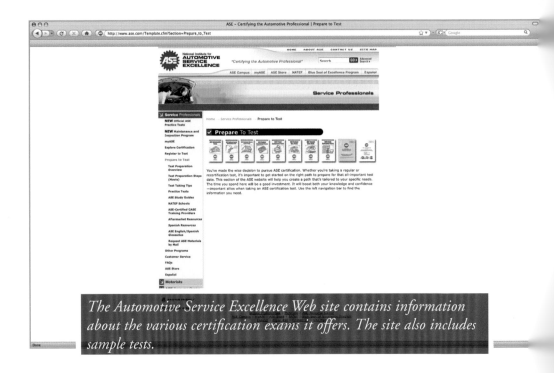

The Automotive Service Excellence Web site contains information about the various certification exams it offers. The site also includes sample tests.

- Engine machinist
- Alternate fuels
- Advanced engine performance specialist
- Medium/heavy truck
- Truck equipment
- School bus
- Transit bus
- Collision repair and refinish
- Damage analysis and estimating
- Parts specialist
- Electronic diesel engine diagnosis
- Undercar specialist

It's not necessary to take these tests to be hired as a technician. All of them are completely voluntary. They are not required by law, but they often are by employers. Those with ASE certification are more likely to get hired, especially by the larger garages and dealerships that typically require it. Those with ASE certification are also likely to get paid more throughout their career. The ASE patches and certification will make someone a more valued employee, a more skilled mechanic, and a more trusted personal service technician.

EXPLORING YOUR EDUCATIONAL OPTIONS

So you've decided the field of automotive mechanics is for you, and you've already explored many of the options that are outlined in the last chapter. You have decided to get further education and practical training before you start searching for your first job. But how do you get started on your education?

There are two basic choices. You can attend community college classes, usually for a period of six to twelve months, or

AN INSIDE LOOK AT THE
ASE CERTIFICATION EXAM

What kind of knowledge is tested on an automotive technician's exam? Here are a few multiple-choice questions taken from *Automotive Technician Certification Test Preparation Manual* (3rd edition), by Don Knowles:

From the "Steering Systems" section of the test:
The steering on a vehicle pulls to the right while driving straight ahead. The cause of this problem could be:
    A. More toe-out on the right rear wheel than on the left rear wheel.
    B. More positive camber on the left front wheel than on the right front wheel.
    C. More toe-out on turns on the left front wheel than on the right front wheel.
    D. More positive caster on the left front wheel than on the right front wheel.
(Correct answer: D)

From the "Brakes" section:
A vehicle experiences brake drag on all four wheels. Technician A says the master cylinder compensating ports may be plugged. Technician B says the rubber cups in the master cylinder may be swollen. Who is correct?
    A. A only.
    B. B only.
    C. Both A and B.
    D. Neither A nor B.
(Correct answer: C)

From the "Operating Systems" section:

All of the following statements about computer-controlled air-conditioning (A/C) system actuator motors are true EXCEPT:

A. Some actuator motors are calibrated automatically in the self-diagnostic mode.

B. A/C system diagnostic trouble codes represent a fault in a specific component.

C. The actuator motor control rods must be calibrated manually on some systems.

D. The actuator motor control rods should only require adjustment after motor replacement or misalignment.

(Correct answer: B)

you can go to a post-secondary (after graduation from high school) vocational school for two years and earn an associate's degree. Both options will offer you a combination of classroom instruction and hands-on experience and practice. They will both have the most up-to-date technical data to teach with, as well as the newest types of diagnostic equipment. An associate's degree program usually combines all of this with additional courses in English, math, and the sciences.

You can find community colleges and vocational schools in your area by searching online. Some of these schools are statewide or even nationwide institutions, with local campuses near you. The Universal Technical Institute, for example, has campuses in Arizona, Pennsylvania, Texas, Florida, and elsewhere. Some Web sites, such as MechanicSchools.com, provide information regarding vocational schools throughout the nation. Bear in mind that technical and vocational colleges are great, but they also cost a lot of money—upwards of

$25,000. Junior colleges are a terrific alternative, and they cost only about $5,000.

In addition to traditional community colleges and technical/vocational schools, some auto manufacturers and dealers offer

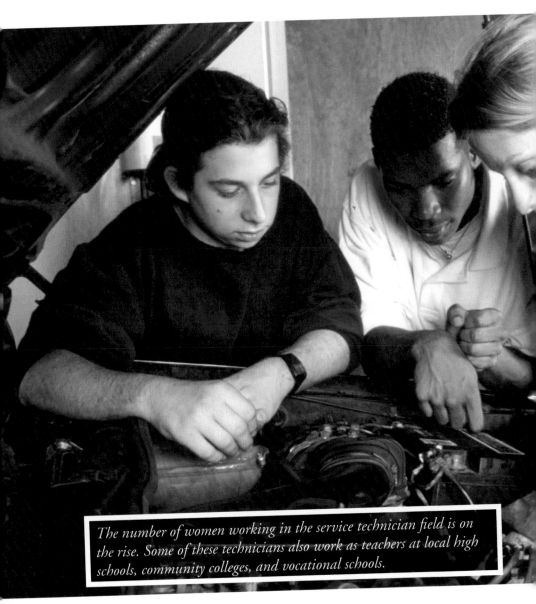

The number of women working in the service technician field is on the rise. Some of these technicians also work as teachers at local high schools, community colleges, and vocational schools.

their own two-year associate's degree programs. Once enrolled, students alternate between working in the dealer's service department and going to school every six to twelve weeks.

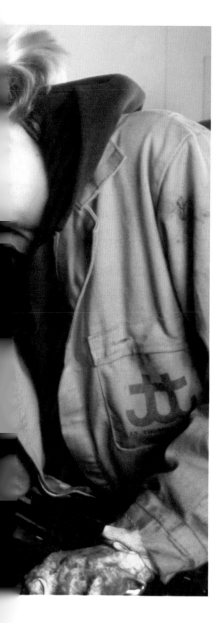

LIFELONG LEARNING ON THE JOB

Once you have completed your education and find your first job, don't think you are finished learning. The automotive industry is constantly changing, and its vehicles are always becoming more complex and high-tech. For this reason, continuing education is absolutely necessary for the technician who wishes to remain knowledgeable and skilled. Employers typically send their technicians to manufacturers' training centers to learn how to repair new model cars or get specific training on repairing individual components. Other times, factory representatives will come to the dealership to present workshops to the technicians.

Experts in the field state that it takes two to five years on the job before veteran mechanics consider newer employees to be fully

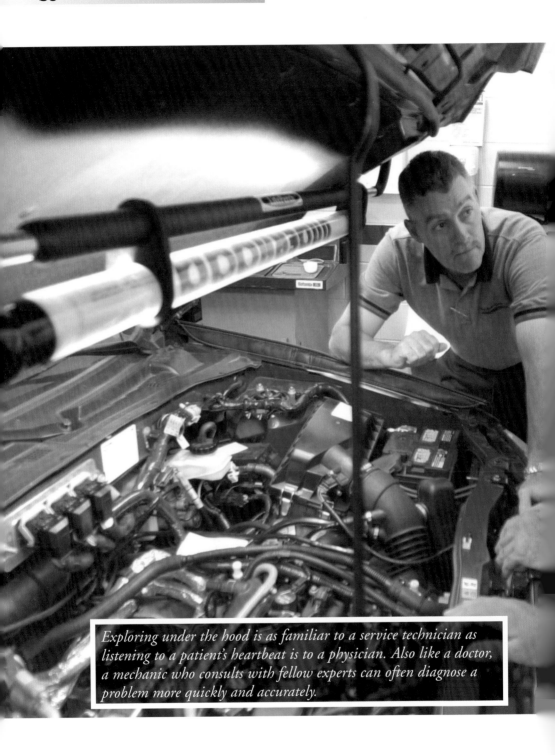

Exploring under the hood is as familiar to a service technician as listening to a patient's heartbeat is to a physician. Also like a doctor, a mechanic who consults with fellow experts can often diagnose a problem more quickly and accurately.

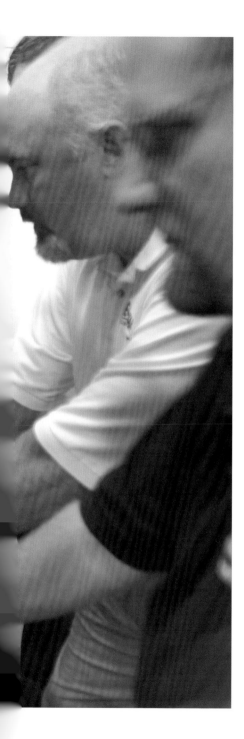

qualified service technicians. It requires one to two additional years to become familiar with every type of car repair. And if you specialize in one particular area, such as transmissions, that can take an additional one to two years to truly master.

When it comes to automotive maintenance and repair, it's important to remember that practice makes perfect. It takes time to develop talent and to gain knowledge and experience in order to become a truly competent and skilled technician. You won't learn these skills quickly, but with time, you can become a valued and respected employee who makes the cars we all drive far safer and more reliable.

What About Women?

Although the vast majority of auto technicians are men, it does not mean that women are unable to do the job. Indeed, a growing number of women are entering the field. In an interview with Bridget Ryan

THE AUTOMOTIVE YOUTH EDUCATIONAL SYSTEMS (AYES)

The AYES is a nationwide partnership between automotive manufacturers, participating dealerships, and more than 350 secondary automotive schools. According to its Web site, it exists to: "Enhance the public image of dealerships and dealership careers, build local partnerships between dealerships and high-quality schools, and foster positive working environments in dealerships." Dealerships today are in competition for qualified employees, not only among themselves, but also among restaurants, mass marketers, other retail outlets, and other professions. Dealerships need to reach out to young people and their parents to explain the challenges and rewards of pursuing a retail automotive career. AYES is helping in this effort by providing how-to ideas and support materials on conducting dealership tours for educators and youngsters, offering job shadowing opportunities, and taking part in career days and career fairs at local schools.

A select number of high school juniors are invited to participate in AYES every year. In addition to their regular school classes, they take additional courses in either basic automotive technology or collision repair and refinishing. They are also instructed in the importance of a positive attitude and teamwork in the workplace. During the summer between their junior and senior years, these students begin internships at local dealerships on a full-time basis. Experienced technicians mentor them carefully. At graduation, students are offered entry-level, full-time jobs.

Snell for *Motor Age* magazine, Lorri Toni, an educator and trainer in automotive tech, said:

> I love being a part of these industries. There is so much opportunity in a myriad of trades and technical careers. It is so unfortunate that neither boys nor girls are aware of these wonderful and challenging options. It is hard to be a pioneer, but it is also very rewarding. I envision a day when women in any career will be just matter-of-fact, and there will not be a need for special articles about our uniqueness! This country cannot meet all the challenges of our rapidly evolving future without the expertise and education of both our men and our women. I am excited about how automotive technology can bring math and science to life! What a wonderful field of knowledge—it is truly a treasure of concepts that can lead to limitless opportunity. My automotive technology degree opened so many doors—some that I am still finding!

The number of female techs may be growing, but acceptance of them is still sometimes lacking. It is not unusual for women to have to deal with issues of discrimination from both their coworkers and their customers. Bonnie Durekson, a service manager, said to *Motor Age*, "There are a lot of men who refuse to talk to me because I am a woman. I've had them tell me that they don't think I was educated enough to answer their questions."

Both Toni and Durekson have advice for other young women who are thinking about pursuing careers in the automotive industry. "Do not try to be a man. Be a woman," advised Toni. "The industry needs your 'softness' and caring nature. Customers appreciate it—and profit and success are based on customer satisfaction." Durekson added, "There will be a lot of hurdles and challenges in our industry, just like in any other. But if you stay positive, work smart, and always focus on the solution, not just the problem, you'll overcome the obstacles."

Michele Winn, a service tech, added in the same interview with *Motor Age*, "Don't give up! Remember that this industry is becoming more focused on electronic and computer skills, not dirty, heavy work. With the changes in technology, shop own-ers realize that the best person for the job may not always be a man. I believe they just want someone intelligent, professional, and qualified! There is a huge shortage of technicians across the country; this is a great time to look for a job."

More information on opportunities for women in the industry can be found through the Institute for Women Auto Mechanics and its Web site (see the "For More Information" section at the back of this book).

chapter 4

THE RIGHT TOOLS FOR THE JOB

Having great dexterity—being "good with your hands"—is an important quality for anyone going into mechanics. Equally important is having the proper hand tools for the profession. The availability and quality of tools are often the main keys to whether a job is slow and frustrating or smooth and efficient.

Tools are certainly one of a mechanic's most essential helpers and greatest investments. Most technicians have a personal set of tools that they have collected over the years. In addition, the place where they work supplies some of the biggest, most complex, and expensive equipment like diagnostic computers, pneumatic drills, hydraulic lifts, and other large power tools.

TOOLS OF THE TRADE

What tools do mechanics use most frequently? In any given day, a mechanic will use enough different hand tools to fill a large toolbox. You should start with the basics, including the following tools and equipment:

- Drain pan
- Gloves
- Rags

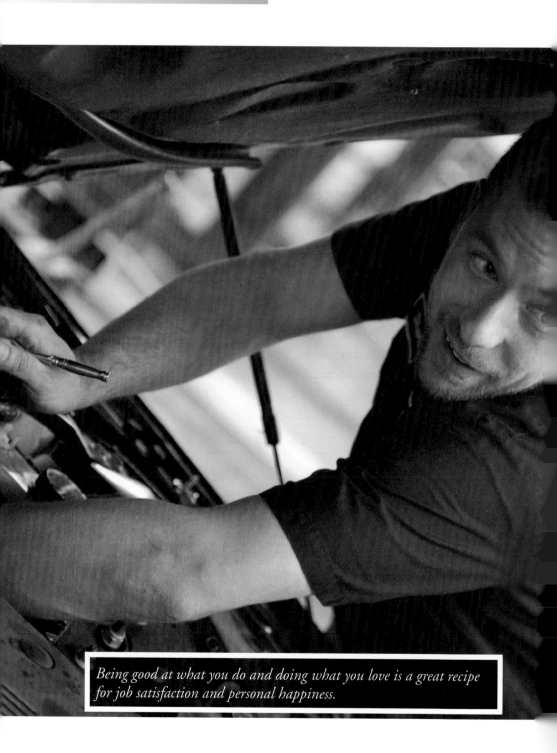

Being good at what you do and doing what you love is a great recipe for job satisfaction and personal happiness.

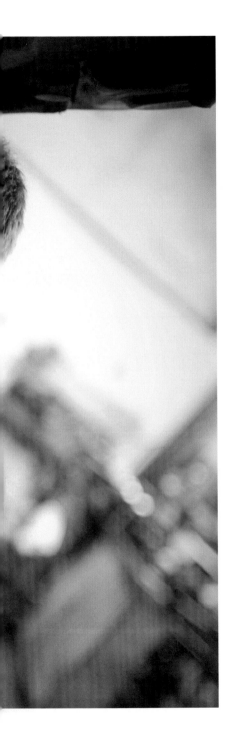

- Safety glasses
- Earplugs
- Funnels
- Screwdrivers
- Wrenches
- Hammers
- Pliers
- Socket sets
- Allen keys
- Wire cutters
- Pry bars
- Wire brushes
- Feeler gauges
- Calipers

Power tools are also essential to a mechanic's daily work. An electric motor, a compressed air motor, or a gasoline engine powers them. The tools can either be portable (hand-held) or stationary. They are typically used for cutting, shaping, drilling, sanding, painting, grinding, and polishing. Some power tools that you might use in automotive work and would probably be provided by your employer include:

- Drill presses
- Bench grinders
- Lathes

The Evolution of Cars, Technicians, and Their Tools

"Cars have become several orders of magnitude more complex than they were just ten years ago. They have become much more advanced in the technology that they harness to last longer, run more efficiently, and perform better than ever before.

"Secondary diagnostic equipment and devices have largely been replaced by a vehicle's onboard computer system. Mechanical systems have almost been completely replaced with high-tech, computer-controlled systems that require a certain skill level in order to access the information to diagnose what is going on. Technicians MUST use computerized scan tools to work on today's vehicles.

"Vehicles, for the most part, still combine gasoline with oxygen and use combustion to generate power. The change is the integration of the computer and ALL of its computing power to control how the vehicle operates. It is often said that the computers in today's vehicles are more complex than the computers from the Apollo missions. The trick is being able to get the diagnostic information from the vehicle computer, determine the root cause of the failure, and repair it."—*Art Jacobsen, CarMD*

"Over the years, the car has become so much more electronic and computer-oriented. You are dealing today with machines that have more computer components than the spaceship that landed on the Moon in 1969. It's an entirely different profession, and the training that's needed is much more extensive, and every year a new model comes out with new technology. So you've got to be really impressed with the young men and women who work on these things."—*Mark Schienberg, president of the Greater New York Automobile Dealers Association (as quoted on InternetAutoGuide.com)*

- Pneumatic wenches
- Air compressors
- Compression gauges
- Welders/flame-cutting equipment
- Jacks
- Hoists

Besides these hand and power tools, you will probably use computerized diagnostic equipment that remains in the dealership or garage where you work. Today, vehicles that come

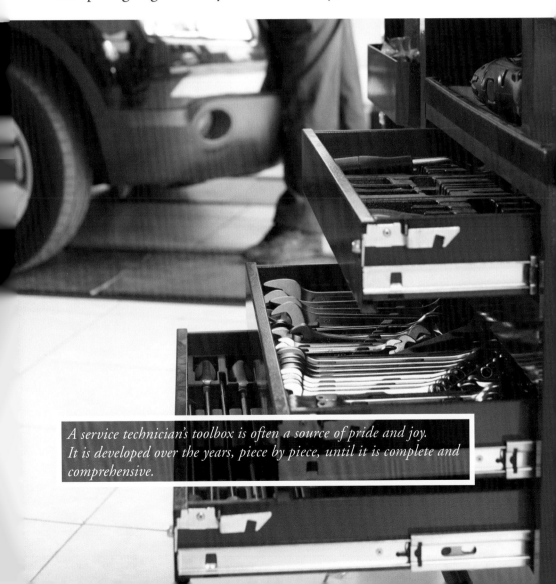

A service technician's toolbox is often a source of pride and joy. It is developed over the years, piece by piece, until it is complete and comprehensive.

into a repair shop are often linked up to computers that test their various systems. A readout compares the test results with a set of benchmark standards issued by the manufacturer. The technician watches for any deviations from the norm. Dealerships and garages get regular updates from car manufacturers about specific car models, their systems, and individual parts to add to their on-site library of technical manuals. They also have access to technical service bulletins and Internet databases. These sources of information provide new technical details, highlight common problems, and explain new maintenance procedures and repair techniques. Computers also help diagnose problems with the high-tech equipment installed in the newest, most modern cars, such as global positioning systems (GPS) and self-parking mechanisms.

An Onboard Technician

As vehicles have become more technologically advanced and computerized, manufacturers have installed a number of computerized self-checks within each model. Most new cars now feature monitors that constantly check systems for proper operation. Some of these monitors are continuous, meaning they run whenever the engine is running. Some of them are noncontinuous, meaning they run through their internal checklists only once per trip.

A number of products also exist to help the owner keep a close eye on how his or her car, van, SUV, or other vehicle is operating. One of the newest is CarMD. It was developed to help drivers know if something is wrong and what to do about it. "CarMD works by tapping into your vehicle's onboard computer system and extracting information about the current operating condition of your vehicle," explains Art Jacobsen, director of business development and the former vice president

FILLING UP ON FRENCH FRIES

One of the most common terms thrown around about vehicles today is "alternative fuels." What exactly qualifies as an alternative fuel? Technically, it is any fuel that is not made from petroleum. Such fuels include:

- Alcohols (ethanol and methanol)
- Electricity (batteries)
- Hydrogen
- Compressed natural gas
- Liquefied natural gas
- Liquids made from coal
- Biodiesel (from plant oil or animal fat)

Ethanol, often known as grain alcohol, is usually made from corn, but sometimes other organic material like rice straw is used. Methanol, known as wood alcohol, is made from coal. It has been used in race cars for decades because it is safer in case of accidental fire. Flexible fuel vehicles have also been developed for consumers. They operate on alcohol, gasoline, or a combination of the two.

Biodiesel fuels, or those made from vegetable oil or animal fat, are slowly developing into a real energy alternative. They are less harmful to the environment and are fairly easy to come by. Some of the most popular types of biodiesel fuel come from either soybeans or the used cooking oil from restaurants. Because this type of fuel is made from plants and animals, it is considered renewable—a definite plus when it comes to often scarce and dwindling energy sources.

The technicians who work on engines powered by one of these alternative fuels must have up-to-date information in order to maintain and repair them.

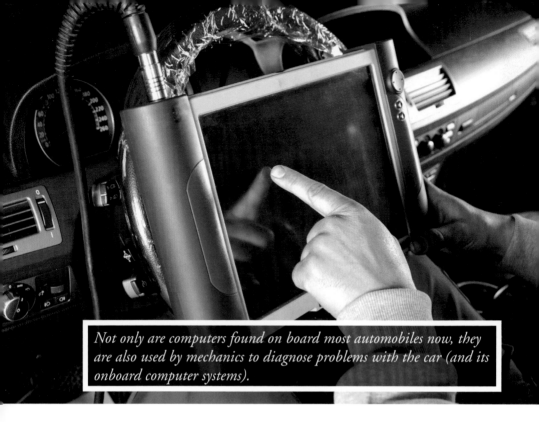

Not only are computers found on board most automobiles now, they are also used by mechanics to diagnose problems with the car (and its onboard computer systems).

of Smart Auto Management. "This information is then cross-referenced with CarMD's massive online database that is built with repair information from ASE master technicians nation-wide. Our database contains real-world solutions to your vehicle's problems."

CarMD allows the driver to take more responsibility for the care and maintenance of his or her vehicle by consulting online with tens of thousands of technicians. It then provides repair suggestions to try at home or to pass along to a local mechanic.

Just as the best surgeon cannot do the job properly without the right scalpel, monitors, and other instruments, neither can the best automotive technician repair any vehicle without specific tools. Knowing what tools are needed for a given job and how to use them is part of what makes a mechanic worth his or her weight in nuts and bolts!

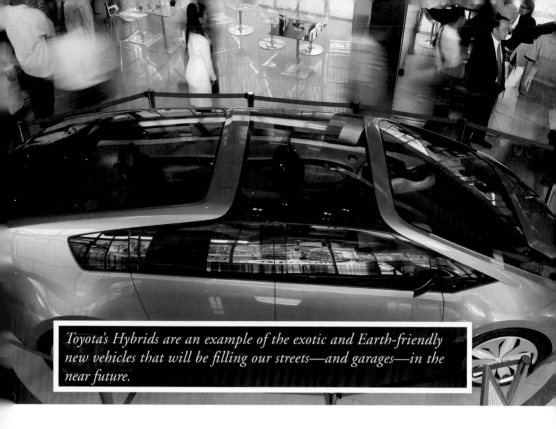

Toyota's Hybrids are an example of the exotic and Earth-friendly new vehicles that will be filling our streets—and garages—in the near future.

TECHNICIANS ADAPT TO ALTERNATIVE FUEL ENGINES

Oil supplies are limited and dwindling, and the burning of fossil fuels contributes to global warming and climate change. For this reason, engineers have been trying to create vehicles that are powered by alternative sources of energy. They have come up with several possibilities.

The engine of a hybrid car is powered by both gasoline and electricity. Usually, these cars have gasoline engines, but rely on an electric motor when speeding up or climbing hills. The motor includes batteries that are continually recharged while you drive. These cars typically get far better gas mileage than regular cars, sometimes getting as much as 68 miles (109 km) per gallon. Examples of hybrids include the Honda Insight, the Honda Civic, and the Toyota Prius.

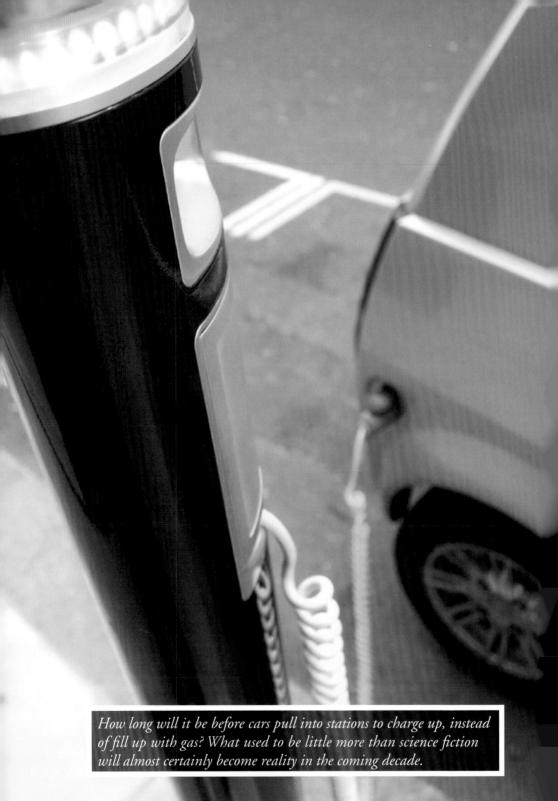

How long will it be before cars pull into stations to charge up, instead of fill up with gas? What used to be little more than science fiction will almost certainly become reality in the coming decade.

Other alternative fuel vehicles being developed are electric vehicles, or EVs. They don't burn gasoline, but they depend on twelve or twenty-four batteries for power. These batteries have to be plugged in each day to recharge. They are designed to go about 200 miles (322 km) between recharging.

Another possibility is the zero emission vehicle, or ZEV. Like spacecraft, these cars feature fuel cells that are powered with pure hydrogen. The fuel cells convert the hydrogen and oxygen into electricity, which, in turn, powers an electric motor.

As vehicles change, so must the automotive technician's skills and knowledge. When vehicle engines make a shift to electricity, hydrogen, or some other new fuel source, the technician will have to adapt to these new technologies as well. It is one of the challenges that make the job so interesting and cutting edge.

chapter 5

ALL-AROUND MECHANICS AND SPECIALISTS

S ome doctors, rather than becoming general practitioners, decide to become specialists in the care of a specific part of the body. In the same way, mechanics can choose to maintain and repair a range of vehicles and makes and models, or they can choose a specialty. It might be only one model of car. It might be only one particular system, such as the exhaust system or transmission. A mechanic might only work on scooters, speedboats, high-performance cars, or all-terrain vehicles (ATVs). The technician might devote himself or herself to a specific make of foreign car. Other technicians may specialize in maintaining a city's fleet of buses, subways, or streetcars.

Areas of specialization can get incredibly specific. For example, there are a handful of experts on the maintenance and repair of air-cooled Volkswagen buses. That is all they work on. Becoming an invaluable specialist or an equally expert generalist—a highly skilled, all-around mechanic—all depends on what interests you the most and what jobs you can find in your area.

Taking the time to read through the eight different examinations given by the ASE might help you determine if you want to specialize in a specific area of vehicle repair and maintenance. Read the questions and study the different divisions within each section. Which appeals to you the most?

THE IMPORTANCE OF BEING WELL ROUNDED

Even if a specific make and model or automotive system appeals to you and you think you might want to specialize in it, it is always wise to develop a broad range of mechanical skills to boost your employability. Tony Molla is vice president of communications for the National Institute for Automotive Service Excellence. He recently pointed out in an interview with Josh Green of MyNC.com how many opportunities there are for good, well-rounded auto technicians:

> Having technical skills can open up quite a few possibilities for those in the automotive industry, but even other industries like Aerospace recognize the value of an

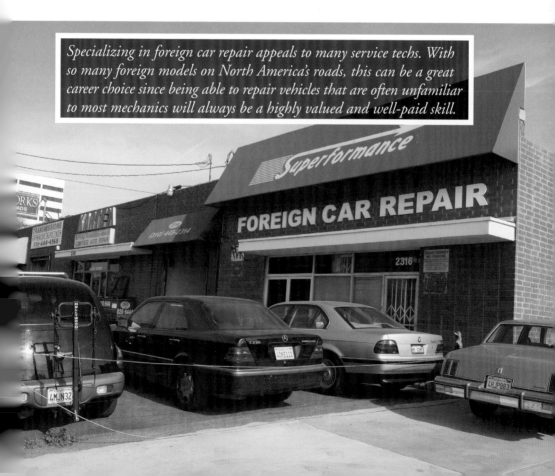

Specializing in foreign car repair appeals to many service techs. With so many foreign models on North America's roads, this can be a great career choice since being able to repair vehicles that are often unfamiliar to most mechanics will always be a highly valued and well-paid skill.

applicant with a technical background. Many parts manufacturers, for example, love to have regional sales representatives with technical backgrounds, since such an individual would not only understand the products and how they are used, they also understand the customer very well. Having a good mastery of electronics, knowing how to use sophisticated test equipment, and being proficient with the use of tools can qualify an individual for a great many things, from shop management to customer service positions. The most obvious opportunities for technicians right now are in the heavy-duty segment, and most of these companies will provide the ongoing training a technician needs to keep their skills sharp and cope with advancing automotive technology.

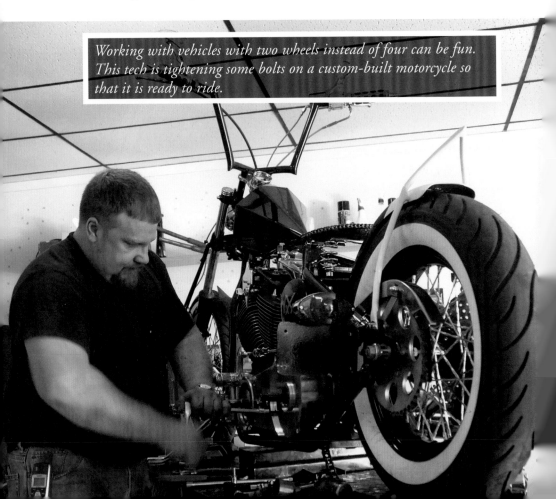

Working with vehicles with two wheels instead of four can be fun. This tech is tightening some bolts on a custom-built motorcycle so that it is ready to ride.

Auto Body Repair

Every single day there are thousands of traffic accidents. Although that is not a happy fact for many, it is what keeps auto body shops in business. If you decide to specialize as an automotive body worker, it will be your job to remove or repair dents, replace damaged parts, and straighten out bent frames and structures.

To do these jobs, you will most likely use equipment like alignment machines powered by hydraulic pressure. They will help you get broken parts back into alignment. Specific benchmark standards will guide you in figuring out where each piece has to go to work properly again. A pneumatic metal-cutting gun may be used to repair body panels, and dents are fixed through a combination of pneumatic hammers, hand prying bars, and hydraulic jacks. Pick hammers and punches can be used to take out the smallest pits. Plastic panels will need to be molded back into place through the use of a hot-air welding gun or simply hot water and lots of patience.

Along with a background in general auto repair, an automotive body worker should be excellent at reading technical manuals and diagrams, as well as measuring and doing quick mathematical figuring. The ASE offers certification in collision repair through four of its exams.

The Art of Motorcycle Maintenance

Another angle to pursue within mechanics is working with two-wheeled and three-wheeled vehicles. There are millions of motorcycles, scooters, mopeds, dirt bikes, and ATVs on the road that need regular maintenance and repair. Some bike mechanics work in garages, while a number of them work for

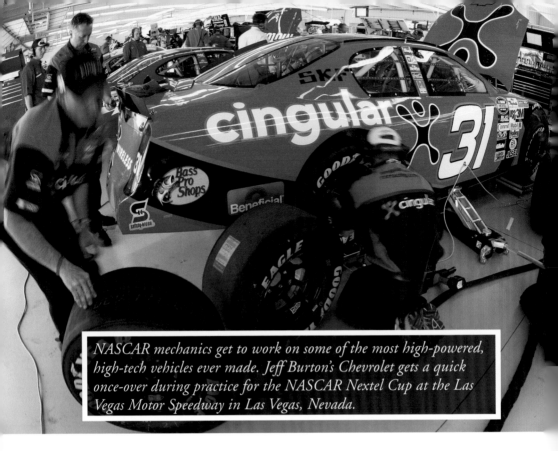

NASCAR mechanics get to work on some of the most high-powered, high-tech vehicles ever made. Jeff Burton's Chevrolet gets a quick once-over during practice for the NASCAR Nextel Cup at the Las Vegas Motor Speedway in Las Vegas, Nevada.

specific dealerships, such as Harley-Davidson, Honda, Yamaha, Suzuki, or Kawasaki.

Classes in motorcycle mechanics include information on repairing forks, transmissions, and drive chains. Students learn how to dismantle engines and replace parts like magnetos, carburetors, and generators. They practice removing cylinder heads and grind valves and hammering out dents and bends, as well as welding tears and breaks. Manual dexterity is extremely important to the motorcycle mechanic because the areas he or she is working within are much smaller and closer together than what are under the hood of a car.

HIGH-PERFORMANCE CARS

Specializing in high-performance cars is another possibility for those interested in a career in mechanics. These cars have a

CERTIFIED AUTO GLASS REPAIR TECHNICIAN PROGRAM

Some automotive technicians choose to specialize in glass repair and replacement. Car windows and windshields get cracked and broken all the time through accidents and collisions. The nationwide Certified Auto Glass Repair Technician Program was partially developed by the National Windshield Repair Association. It measures a technician's abilities through a computerized exam given at testing centers throughout North America.

To be certified, a technician has to have participated in the auto glass business for at least six months and have performed at least two hundred repairs. Or the candidate must have completed an auto glass repair training program and have performed more than two hundred repairs. Typically, the technicians who are certified will include auto glass repair technicians, auto glass technicians, collision repair technicians, and vehicle service dealers. Once the exam is passed, the technician is given a wallet identification card, a uniform patch, and a certificate. The certification has to be renewed every three years.

Training for those interested in earning their certification is provided by a number of different organizations, including the National Glass Association, the Carlite Auto Glass Technicians School, the Automotive Glass Consultants, and the Auto Glass Technical Institute.

great deal of power relative to their overall weight. Sometimes they are thought to be the same as sports cars, but there are subtle differences. High-performance cars have extremely powerful engines and are designed not for the road but for the

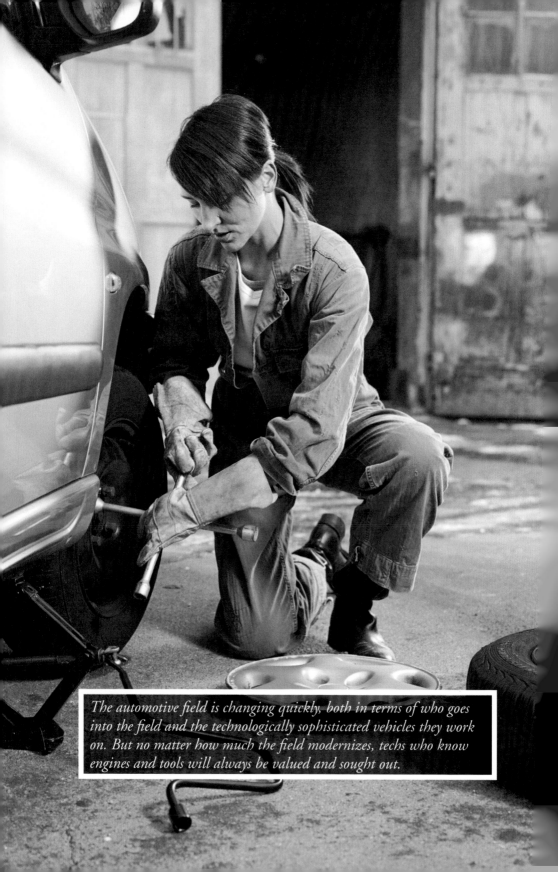

The automotive field is changing quickly, both in terms of who goes into the field and the technologically sophisticated vehicles they work on. But no matter how much the field modernizes, techs who know engines and tools will always be valued and sought out.

racetrack. They can go extremely fast without losing control. Because of this, their structure and engines are often somewhat different than those of the typical passenger car. This means specialized mechanics are needed to work on them.

High-performance car specialists require specific training to make sure the vehicle is reliable even when placed under severe stress. To do so, they frequently use engine analyzers, handheld scanners, and computerized diagnostic equipment. Not only do these technicians need to understand every aspect of the vehicles they are working on, but they also have to learn the tricks to getting every ounce of performance out of the race cars. The drivers' livelihoods—and lives—depend on it.

SOMETHING FOR EVERYONE

With the immense diversity found in the world of automotive technology, there truly is something for everyone. Whether you want to focus on vehicles small or large, vintage or new, American or foreign, transmissions or auto body, general or specialized, ample opportunities are there for you. And chances are, a job opening is as close as your local classified want ads.

chapter 6

OTHER VEHICLES, OTHER ENGINES

C ars, vans, trucks, and SUVs are only some of the vehicles within the field of mechanics that you can work on and explore. Perhaps you would like to work with even larger machines than these.

For example, if you enjoy working with the bigger, more powerful machines, a career maintaining and repairing heavy vehicles and mobile equipment may be a perfect choice for you. These are the vehicles that are used in construction, agriculture, heavy industry, freight and shipping, and the railroads. Technicians repair, replace, clean, lubricate, and maintain heavy equipment. This can include tractors, buses, combines, road graders, cranes, bulldozers, and rail cars. Since many of these machines use hydraulics, technicians must learn how to deal with fluid leaks, ruptured hoses, and worn-out gaskets. Many of the engines used in such large equipment, as well as in trucks, trains, and buses, are diesel engines. Working on them requires additional training.

The same skills and interests that brought you to the field of mechanics can take you in several other exciting directions as well. Some possibilities include marine mechanics, avionics, and small-engine repair. Working on these nonautomotive vehicles can be both fascinating and lucrative. The work can take you to interesting places, like marinas, aircraft carriers,

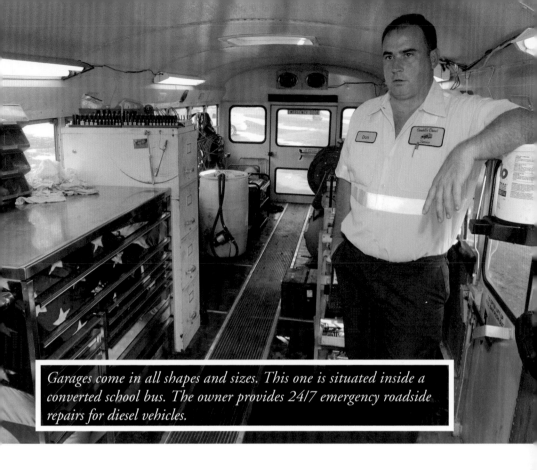

Garages come in all shapes and sizes. This one is situated inside a converted school bus. The owner provides 24/7 emergency roadside repairs for diesel vehicles.

and rocket launchpads. And because these machines are often so crucial to commerce and defense, the pay is great.

OUT ON THE WATER

There are more than 12.8 million recreational boats cruising the waters of the country's lakes, rivers, and oceans. Marine or motorboat mechanics are needed to maintain and service all of them. Inboard motors are usually found on large boats like cabin cruisers, cargo ships, ferries, oil tankers, submarines, and commercial fishing boats.

Because boats are so big, repairs are typically performed by trained mechanics who go to the docks, shipyards, and marinas to work on them. Outboard engines, on the other hand, are

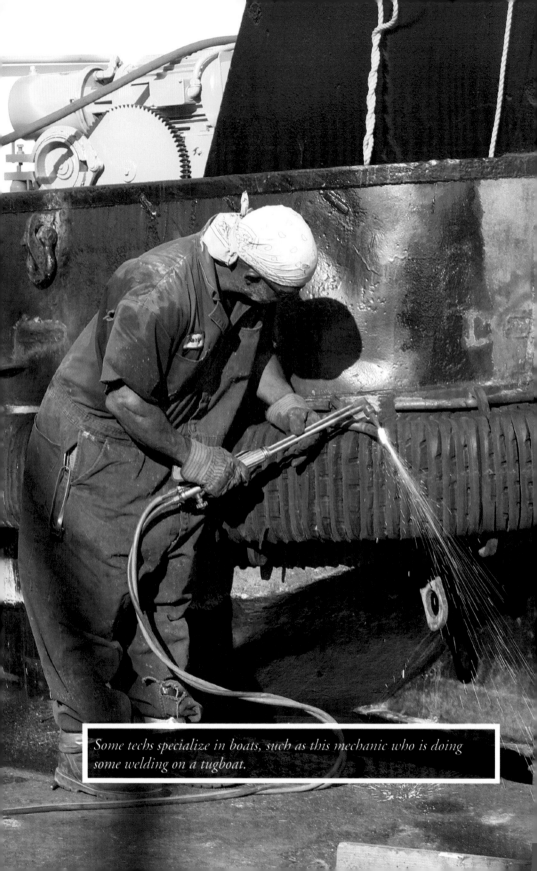

Some techs specialize in boats, such as this mechanic who is doing some welding on a tugboat.

typically found on small boats, Jet Skis, yachts, and other motorized watercraft. Repairs on these lighter craft are done in garages because the smaller engines can be brought in and left behind. Technicians work not only on engines, but also on propellers, plumbing, and steering mechanisms. On larger ships, they may also work on air-conditioning and refrigeration

IS THE AUTO TECH INDUSTRY REALLY RECESSION-PROOF?

"It's probably more accurate to say it's recession-resistant. However, most of our independent repair shops are reporting increased sales as more consumers choose to maintain their older (and often paid-for) vehicle, rather than commit to five- or six-years' worth of car payments for something new. Maintaining a good used vehicle is usually a very cost-effective option, with even comprehensive repair bills only representing one or two car payments. Add to this the fact that, for most Americans, our personal vehicles are our mass-transit system, which millions of us rely on to get to work, school, the grocery store, etc."—*Tony Molla, vice president of communications for the National Institute for Automotive Service Excellence, as quoted in Josh Green's article "The Recession-Resistant Job?"*

"Automotive testing and repair is a great field to get into. We rely on our vehicles to get us safely from [point] A to B on a daily basis. Being without your vehicle is a huge problem most people cannot tolerate for extended periods of time. With that being said, and combining it with the fact that people are driving their vehicles for much longer today, the future for automotive repair certainly looks bright."—*Art Jacobsen, CarMD* systems. Common maintenance procedures include checking parts for safety; replacing wiring; inspecting pumps, gears, and rings; and realigning the steering.

Depending on where you live, repair and maintenance of marine craft can be seasonal work, so it may be difficult to find enough to do during the fall and winter months. Living near resort areas or coastal regions, where the weather allows for boating year-round, can be the best choice. You may work directly for a marina or for a dealership or boat manufacturer. No matter where you work, you will most likely spend a great deal of time out in the sun and near the water—a great job perk.

Marine mechanics can go to professional technical schools to learn the business and enter two-year programs to earn an associate's degree.

UP IN THE AIR

Another type of specialization you might want to explore is avionics, or aircraft mechanics. Avionics programs are offered by 170 schools across the country. The Federal Aviation Administration (FAA) has certified each of them. The programs range in length from eighteen months to four years.

The field of avionics includes everything from propeller-driven and jet engine commercial passenger planes to helicopters, fighters, and bombers. Aircraft mechanics do a variety of jobs. These include inspecting, maintaining, and repairing aircraft engines, landing gear, instruments, pressurized sections, accessory brakes, valves, pumps, and air-conditioning systems. They check for cracks in the engine, fuselage, wings, and tail using X-rays and magnetic inspection.

Like any qualified mechanic, avionics technicians repair and replace worn and/or defective parts. They measure tension on the aircraft's control cables. They work on the craft's

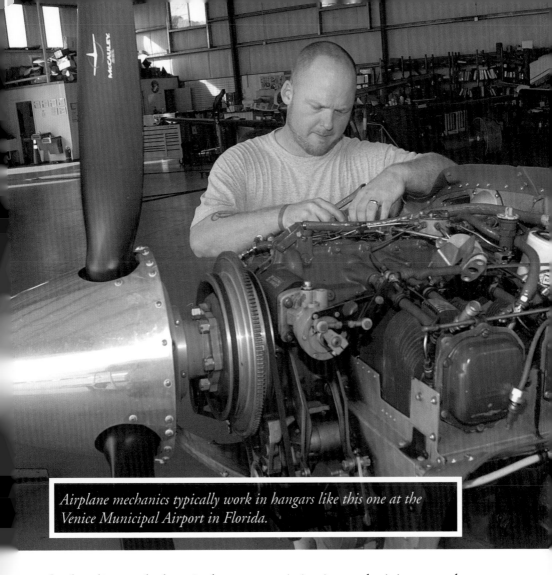

Airplane mechanics typically work in hangars like this one at the Venice Municipal Airport in Florida.

hydraulics and electrical systems. Avionics technicians work on virtually anything that is involved in both navigation and communication on aircraft, including the weather radar systems. In addition, these mechanics also keep very detailed maintenance records.

SMALL BUT POWERFUL

A third common type of mechanics that you can get involved in is working with small engines. Technicians are needed to

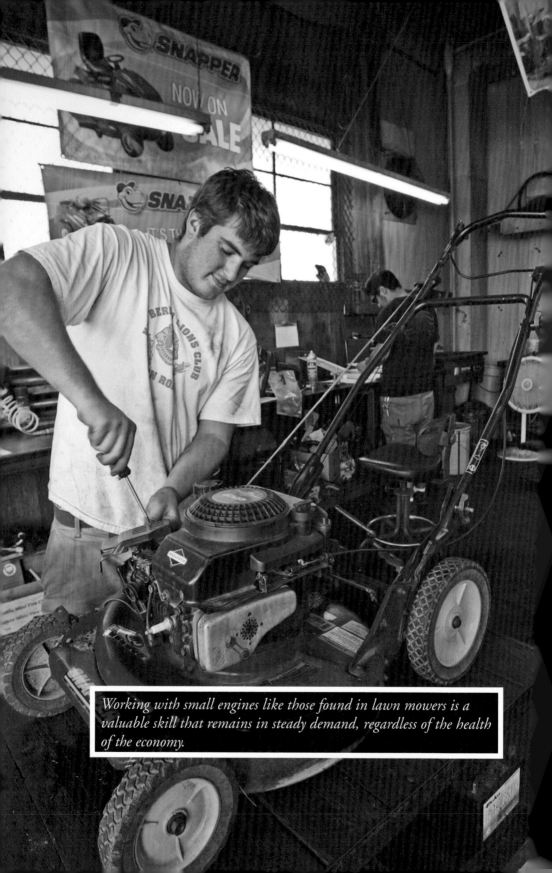

Working with small engines like those found in lawn mowers is a valuable skill that remains in steady demand, regardless of the health of the economy.

repair and service power equipment like chain saws, edge trimmers, lawn mowers, go-carts, portable generators, snowblowers, and snowmobiles. Typically, a technician specializes in a particular type of equipment.

Technicians who choose this field learn how to do everything from replacing a single part to performing a complete overhaul of the equipment. In the case of a ride-on lawn mower or go-cart, they may inspect and clean the engine, brakes, fuel injection systems, plugs, and carburetors, following a set checklist of what needs to be examined. Other times, they perform regular maintenance service to ensure that the machine is working at peak performance. Although most mechanics rely on hand tools for this job, some may also use more complex tools. These can include compression gauges, ammeters, voltmeters, and computerized engine analyzers.

A GROWING NEED

According to the Bureau of Labor Statistics, the auto industry will need approximately thirty-five thousand new technicians every year through 2016. For the past few years, the number of students going into the field has been dropping. This has been the case even though the field has been expanding and potential incomes have been rising steadily. "The business of being an auto mechanic has been . . . depicted as a dirty, greasy kind of job. The truth today is it's a very high-tech, good-paying job. There is a demand and a shortage," says Michael Calkins, manager of AAA's auto repair division, in an interview published in *USA Today*. "People who come out of school have jobs waiting for them."

Brian Miller, chairman of the Greater New York Automobile Dealers Association, agrees. In an interview with the *New York Daily News*, he says, "A guy starting out as an auto technician can make fifty grand [$50,000] in the first year. It can go up to $150,000. It's really a wide-open field. There's a shortage of technicians, and it's not like the old days where mechanics didn't make a whole lot. They can make great money."

Vehicles are evolving to keep pace with a technologically advancing world, dwindling fuel supplies, and potential new energy sources. Highly skilled automotive technicians who can not only keep up with these changes, but also race ahead to understand what tomorrow's needs might be and how the new machines will work will be highly valued. Becoming an automotive technician gives you the chance to expand and hone your talents while making each vehicle you work on safer and better. And you get paid well for doing something you love and are great at. It's a win-win situation for everyone!

glossary

alignment The proper adjustment of the components of a machine.

ammeter An instrument that measures electric current.

avionics The science and technology of the development and use of electrical and electronic devices in aviation.

biodiesel fuel Fuel made from vegetable oil or animal fat.

calipers An instrument for measuring thicknesses or distances between surfaces.

carburetor A device for mixing fuel with air, as in an internal combustion engine.

certification The state of being certified or officially endorsed.

deviation Departure from a standard or norm.

dexterity Skill in using one's hands.

diagnostics A message produced by a computer diagnosing a problem with the system.

discrimination Treatment in favor of or against a person based on the group, class, or category to which that person belongs, rather than on individual merit.

domestic Made in one's own country, in the case of manufactured goods like cars.

fraud Intentional deception for the purpose of profit or gain.

gasket A rubber, metal, or rope ring placed around a joint or piston.

hoist An apparatus for hoisting or lifting something up into the air.

hybrid A blending of two things.

hydraulic Operated or moved by water or other liquids in motion.

magneto A small electric generator often used with internal combustion engines.

marina A boat basin offering service for small watercraft.

petroleum An oily, thick, dark liquid obtained by drilling into the earth and ocean floor and used as fuel.

pneumatic Operated by air or by the pressure of air.

renewable Pertaining to something that can be replaced or reused.

schematic A diagram, plan, or drawing.

suspension The arrangement of springs, shock absorbers, hangers, etc., in an automobile or other vehicle.

transmission Transference of force between machines or mechanisms, often with changes of torque and speed.

vocational Pertaining to an occupation or a trade.

voltmeter An instrument for measuring the electrical potential difference between two points in an electric circuit.

for more information

Accrediting Commission of Career Schools and Colleges of
    Technology (ACCSCT)
2101 Wilson Boulevard, Suite 302
Arlington, VA 22201
(703) 247-4212
Web site: http://oedb.org/accreditation-agencies/accsct
The ACCSCT promotes enhanced opportunities for students
    by establishing, sustaining, and enforcing valid standards
    and practices that contribute to the development of a
    highly trained and competitive workforce through quality,
    career-oriented education.

Automotive Careers Today (ART)
8400 Westpark Drive, #2
McLean, VA 22012
Web site: http://www.autocareerstoday.net
ART, a coalition of major automobile manufacturers and
    dealer organizations, works to promote a better under-
    standing of the retail side of the automotive industry and
    build stronger customer relationships through shared
    research and development programs.

Automotive Youth Education System (AYES)
100 West Big Beaver, Suite 300
Troy, MI 48084
(888) 339-2937
Web site: https://www.ayes.org
The AYES is a partnership of auto manufacturers, dealerships,
    and secondary automotive programs that encourages

young people to consider careers in retail automotive service and prepare them for entry-level positions or advanced studies in automotive technology.

Bureau of Labor Statistics (BLS)
2 Massachusetts Avenue NE
Washington, DC 20212-0001
(202) 691-5200
Web site: http://www.bls.gov
The BLS is an independent national statistical agency that collects, processes, analyzes, and disseminates essential statistical data to the American public, the U.S. Congress, other federal agencies, state and local governments, business, and labor.

Institute for Women Auto Mechanics
244 Fifth Avenue, #G205
New York, NY 10001-7604
(917) 254-1772
Web site: http://theinstitute4womenautomechanics.com
Among other things, the Institute for Women Auto Mechanics teaches women how to prevent costly automotive breakdowns and save money by doing their own auto repairs.

National Automotive Technology Education
    Foundation (NATEF)
101 Blue Seal Drive, Suite 101
Leesburg, VA 20175
(703) 669-6650
Web site: http://www.natef.org
The NATEF is a nonprofit organization that evaluates technician-training programs against standards developed

by the auto industry and recommends qualifying programs for certification by ASE, the National Institute for Automotive Service Excellence.

National Institute for Automotive Service Excellence (ASE)
101 Blue Seal Drive SE, Suite 101
Leesburg, VA 20175
(888) 273-8378
Web site: http://www.ase.com
The mission of the ASE is to improve the quality of vehicle repair and service through the testing and certification of repair and service professionals. About four hundred thousand professionals hold current certifications.

WEB SITES

Due to the changing nature of Internet links, Rosen Publishing has developed an online list of Web sites related to the subject of this book. This site is updated regularly. Please use this link to access the list:

http://www.rosenlinks.com/ecar/mech

for further reading

Borg, Kevin L. *Auto Mechanics: Technology and Expertise in Twentieth Century America* (Studies in Industry and Society). Baltimore, MD: Johns Hopkins University Press, 2007.

Brand, Paul. *How to Repair Your Car* (Motorbooks Workshop). Minneapolis, MN: Motorbooks, 2006.

Jozefowicz, Chris. *Auto Technician* (Cool Careers). Strongsville, OH: Gareth Stevens, 2009.

Lynn, Vyvyan, and Tony Molla. *The Complete Idiot's Guide to Auto Repair*. New York, NY: Penguin, 2007.

Robert Bosch GmbH. *Automotive Electrics and Automotive Electronics*. Hoboken, NJ: Wiley, 2007.

Robert Bosch GmbH. *Automotive Handbook*. 7th ed. Hoboken, NJ: Wiley, 2007.

Robert Bosch GmbH. *Diesel-Engine Management*. Hoboken, NJ: Wiley, 2006.

Robert Bosch GmbH. *Gasoline-Engine Management*. Hoboken, NJ: Wiley, 2006.

Robert Bosch GmbH. *Safety, Comfort, and Convenience Systems*. Hoboken, NJ: Wiley, 2007.

Sclar, Deanna. *Auto Repair for Dummies*. Hoboken, NJ: Wiley, 2009.

Stockel, Martin T., and Chris Johanson. *Auto Fundamentals*. Tinley Park, IL: Goodheart-Willcox Co., 2005.

Stockel, Martin T., and Chris Johanson. *Auto Fundamentals Workbook*. Tinley Park, IL: Goodheart-Willcox Co., 2005.

Thompson, Lisa. *Pop the Hood: Have You Got What It Takes to Be an Auto Technician?* Minneapolis, MN: Compass Point Books, 2008.

Weintraub, Aileen. *Auto Mechanic*. New York, NY: Children's Press, 2004.

bibliography

Borg, Kevin. *Auto Mechanics: Technology and Expertise in Twentieth Century America*. Baltimore, MD: Johns Hopkins University Press, 2007.

CAGT Exam Secrets Test Prep Team. *Certified Auto Glass Technician Exam Secrets Study Guide*. Beaumont, TX: Mometrix Media LLC, 2009.

Carte, Sharon Silke. "Auto Repair Programs Crank Up Recruitment." *Motor Age*, February 15, 2006. Retrieved September 2009 (http://www.womentechworld.org/bios/ auto/articles/motor.htm).

Caruso, Steve. Interview with author via telephone. September 25, 2009.

Dorries, Elisabeth H. *Automotive Engine Repair and Rebuilding* (Today's Technician). 3rd ed. Florence, KY: Delmar Cengage Learning, 2005.

Duffy, James E. *Auto Body Repair Technology*. Florence, KY: Delmar Cengage Learning, 2008.

Duffy, James E. *Collision Repair Fundamentals*. Florence, KY: Delmar Cengage Learning, 2007.

Green, Josh. "The Recession-Resistant Job?" MyHC.com, September 29, 2009. Retrieved October 2009 (http:// wake.mync.com/site/wake/news/story/42278/ the-recession-resistant-job).

InternetAutoGuide.com. "Future of Auto Mechanic's Salary Looking Bright." August 19, 2008. Retrieved September 2009 (http://blogs.internetautoguide.com/6287325/ industry-news/future-of-auto-mechanics-salary-looking- bright/index.html).

Jacobsen, Art. Interview with author via e-mail. September 26, 2009.

Knowles, Don. *Automotive Technician Certification Test Preparation Manual.* 3rd ed. Florence, KY: Delmar Cengage Learning, 2007.

Max, Josh. "Auto Mechanics Prosper Amid Slow Car Sales." *New York Daily News*, August 18, 2008. Retrieved September 2009 (http://www.nydailynews.com/autos/2008/08/18/2008-08-18_auto_mechanics_prosper_amid_slow_car_sal.html).

Parks, Dennis W. *The Complete Guide to Auto Body Repair* (Motorbooks Workshop). Minneapolis, MN: Motorbooks, 2008.

Snell, Bridget Ryan. "Wearing Her Moxie on Her Sleeve." *Motor Age*, January 2001. Retrieved September 2009 (http://www.womentechworld.org/bios/auto/articles/motor.htm).

Thomas, Alfred M., and Michael Jund. *Collision Repair and Refinishing: A Fundamental Course for Technicians.* Florence, KY: Delmar Cengage Learning, 2009.

Uhrina, Paul, and James E. Duffy. *Auto Body Repair Technology.* 4th ed. Florence, KY: Cengage Learning, 2003.

Vidler, Doug. *Automotive Engine Performance* (Today's Technician). 3rd ed. Florence, KY: Delmar Cengage Learning, 2003.

index

ABOUT THE AUTHOR

Tamra B. Orr is the author of dozens of books for young readers, including many titles relating to science, technology, and careers. She has won several awards for her books. Orr loves being an author because it gives her a chance to learn more about the world every day. She lives in the Pacific Northwest with her husband, children, cat, and dog. She makes sure her children have read every single one of her books.

PHOTO CREDITS

Cover (left) © www.istockphoto.com/Jason Lugo; cover (background), pp. 1, 6, 48 © www.istockphoto.com; p. 4 © www.istockphoto.com/Nathan Gleave; p. 9 © www.istockphoto.com/Lisa Young; p. 11 © Vito Palmisano/Getty Images; pp. 12–13 © www.istockphoto.com/Dr. Heinz Linke; pp. 14, 36–37, 54, 61, 65 © AP Images; p. 15 © www.istockphoto.com/Gene Chutka; pp. 20–21 © Spencer Grant/Photo Edit; p. 22 © Cleve Bryant/Photo Edit; pp. 26–27 © Mercer County Community College; pp. 29, 30 © ASE; pp. 34–35 © Michael Newman/Photo Edit; pp. 42–43 © www.istockphoto.com/William Britten; p. 45 © www.istockphoto.com/Diego Cervo; p. 49 © Saeed Khan/AFP/Getty Images; p. 50 © www.istockphoto.com/Lasse Kristensen; p. 53 © Colin Young-Wolff/Photo Edit; p. 56 © Darrell Ingham/Getty Images; p. 58 © Erik Dreyer/Getty Images; p. 62 © www.istockphoto.com/Glen Jones; p. 66 © Karen Sherlock/MCT/Landov.

Designer: Matthew Cauli; Photo Researcher: Marty Levick